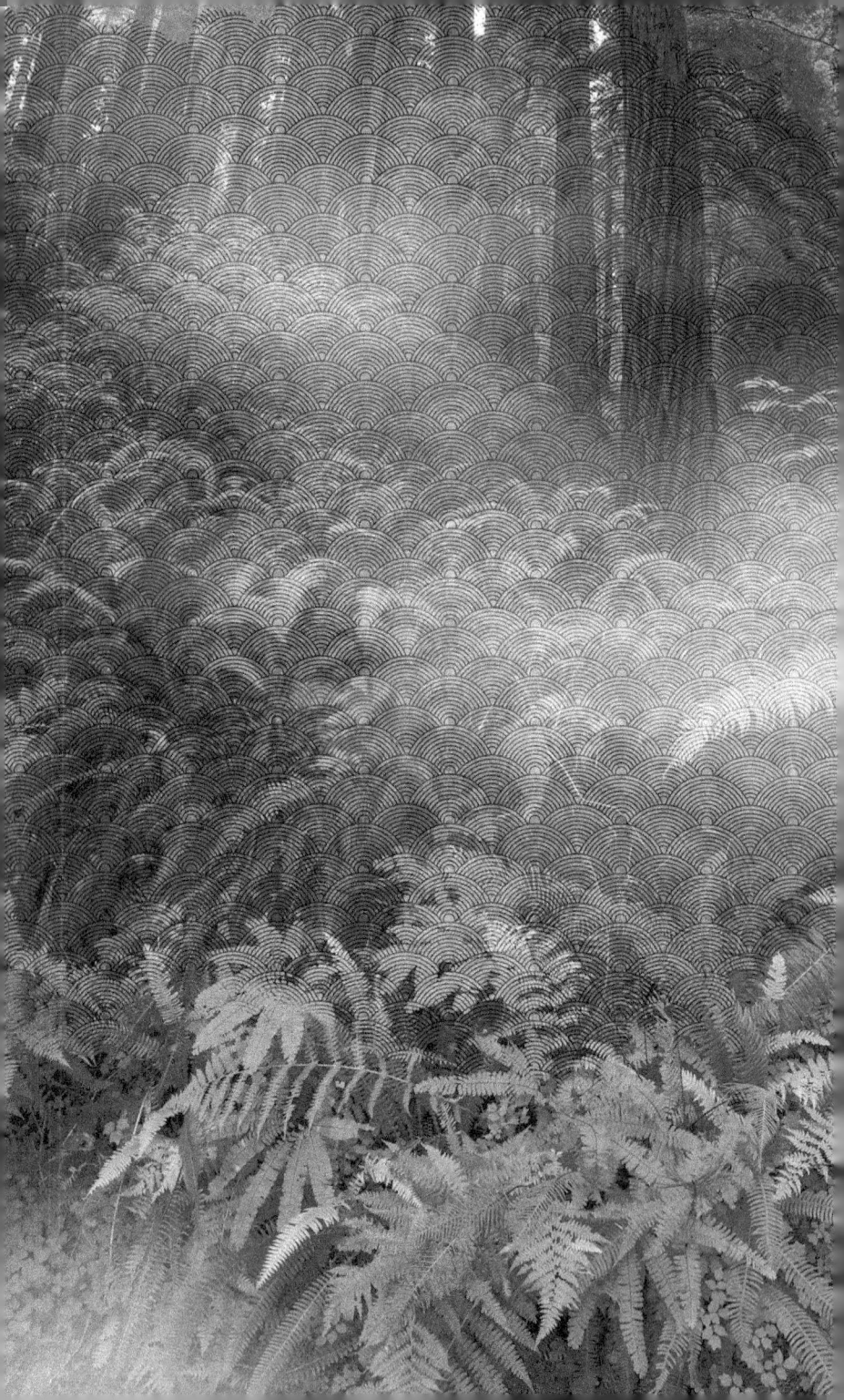

The Evolve Restoration Series
by Beth Alderman, MD, MPH

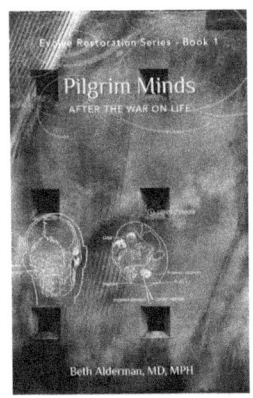

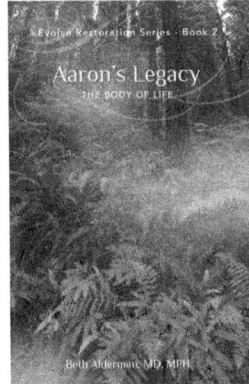

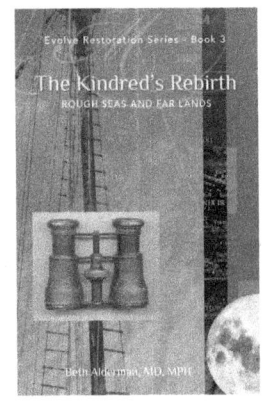

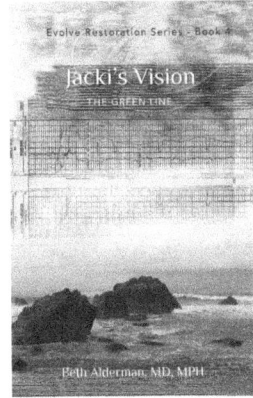

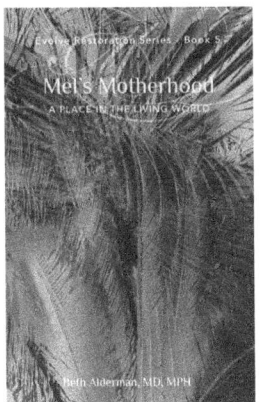

Aaron's Legacy

THE BODY OF LIFE

Book Two of the
Evolve Restoration Series

Beth Alderman MD, MPH

FUTURE MEDICINE LLC • ASHLAND, OREGON

Aaron's Legacy: The Body of Life
by Beth Alderman MD, MPH
© 2019 Beth Alderman
www.LivingFutureBooks.com
For related online courses visit
www.LivingFutureCourses.com

Editor: Julie Clayton
Cover Art: BruceBayard.com
Book Design: BookSavvyStudio.com

Library of Congress Control Number: 2019903854
ISBN: 978-1-7321110-6-6
First Edition
Printed in the United States of America

Contents

1   Pea's Legacy 1

2   Melissa's Legacy 15

3   Coming of Age 31

4   Colette's Legacy 49

5   Disruptors 63

6   Reggie's Legacy 89

7   Entanglement 113

8   Metamorphs 147

9   Eden 173

10   Origin Rite 189

11   God-wrestling 203

12   Discovery 217

13   Kindred 229

Acknowledgments 247

About the Author 249

Books by Beth Alderman 251

To Eva and Bryan

Be not afeard. The isle is full of noises,
Sounds, and sweet airs that give delight and hurt not.
Sometimes a thousand twangling instruments
Will hum about mine ears, and sometime voices
That, if I then had waked after long sleep,
Will make me sleep again. And then, in dreaming,
The clouds methought would open and show riches
Ready to drop upon me, that I waked
I cried to dream again.

— William Shakespeare as Caliban

1

Pea's Legacy

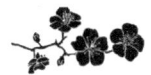

Aaron is sitting stage left with Parvati, Sarah, Rafa, Yukie, John, and Gina, glad that he did not delay the enactments any longer. Rafa's choice of vocation was quick, and Doug's efforts to help her have drawn both pilgrims deep into the Saltspring Research Station, its history, and his family's role in it. They are both ready to explore Pea's legacy. Taking a deep breath, he looks curiously around the theater, which is brightened by the morning light and darkened by the forest. He realizes that he does not know what to expect.

The back benches of the audience oval stand empty. Sarah begins the enactment on time with an introduction of her college friendship group, and then of Aaron's family. He is surprised by the sophisticated projection and soundscape orchestrated from a platform behind the cycle block, where Björn's Viking hair appears and disappears as he operates the lights and sounds. Birds respond from the trees. So far, everything is mundane and familiar.

Aaron finds himself lulled into relaxation and lifted into a fertile care state by the community members on stage. The action begins with an encounter between his mother and her friend Pea that must have taken place before he was born. He is still trying to orient himself when members of the community pause the action to comment on or to question the actors and others on stage. At first, he is annoyed and then overwhelmed, but is surprised to notice that the audience remains unperturbed and attentive. This living dialogue with their history is what they expect. Aaron strains to track the interaction as well as the action, and after a time recognizes that it is like reading aloud and pausing to talk about a text—like Talmud study, in which he reads and reconciles the scripture and its commentaries.

He soon grasps that Leilani and Siobhan, the proponents of intentional human breeding who have been agitating against Sarah, are Pea's granddaughters through Rose. He attended Pea's and Rose's funerals years ago, but does not recall the mourners. Sarah mentions that she invited Jerome's grandson, called Jerbeau, to the next enactment. Aaron remembers Jerome and his son. Feeling the living past enveloping him, Aaron finally grasps Sarah's relation to life in time—to biological time—and recognizes that the legacy transmission and project will give him a chance to come to terms with the whole of his life, and so to make the best of it as he engages it to create his legacy.

Aaron also grasps that the story is about the era when Pea and his mother recognized the peril of environmental contamination, as well as new and mysterious patterns of illness, but had no way to put the two together.

As the performance guilder playing Pea enacts the first stage of the outbreak investigation that was her last as a medical detective, John whispers in Sarah's ear. Sarah calls, "Stop!"

The actors freeze as if they are playing one, two, three, red light. The actor seated behind the desk holds his bolo tie at an awkward angle, and Aaron's wrist aches just looking at him. Sarah raises her eyebrows and nods to John, who says, "This office set is inaccurate. Around this time, a man like this might have put on some background music at a very low volume, but he wouldn't have had a television in his office or done his own programming. Just a few years before this, Missy and I had acquired our first personal computers for word processing and presentations, and begun to use the Internet for email. A man of his age would have delegated everything but control, and would have learned to type or to use personal devices much later, probably to connect with his kids or grandkids."

This slipped by Aaron, who was distracted by an intrusive jingle that Parvarti chose from an archived program interrupted by commercial messages. Aaron can hardly believe that he once listened to point-source media willingly and eagerly, and took it personally. He remembers when separation from an electronic device could throw him into a terrible state.

Meanwhile, Sarah calls to the audience, "How many agree with John?" Hands go up hesitantly. The house lights go up, and Sarah waits. When three quarters of the audience members have raised their hands, she says, "Good!"

She then looks at Parvati, who says, "We wanted to convey the way that late moderns were constantly bombarded by images and phrases that drew at least a part of their attention and divided them from experience. They were more likely to embody commercial memes and to purchase products that they didn't want or need than they were to address their most urgent and obvious problems. They were over-stimulated, confounded, and conditioned to look to media for direction. We chose to convey that by bringing into the workplace the influences that they met at home."

John says, "That makes sense. What may be missing is that

people went to the office to get away from that. My office—or lab—became my temple. Work remains my sanctuary to this day."

"Mea culpa," Doug calls out. "My companies proliferated e-devices like rats did fleas. But like John said, that came later. And we know it, so what gives?"

Parvati laughs. "Artistic license. We wanted to convey the continual bombardment of the unconscious by unwanted conditioning."

John interjects, "I would add that when Missy and Pea and I were in medical school, only the oldest professors could still teach by anecdote. Living memory was disappearing."

Parvati smiles and says, with a glance at Yukie, "There you have it. Late moderns were forgetting what they knew and failing to replace it with what they could glean from embodied experience. Those of you who have trouble forgiving the ancestors may find it useful to experience the continual intrusion of irrelevant, manipulative, or carelessly malicious memes."

Sarah looks at Aaron, who only says, "It takes me back."

With no other comments, Sarah calls out, "Go!"

As the Connie character bulldozes straight through bureaucratic obstacles, Aaron finds that he does not recognize her. "I don't think they have her," Aaron says to Parvati.

Parvati calls out, "Connie!"

The actress playing Connie pivots toward Aaron and exclaims, "Don't interrupt me! You don't know me! You aren't born yet!"

Aaron startles, aghast, and says, 'You were the kindest and most loving of all my mother's friends."

A tall, beautiful woman in the audience stands. Elaborately

groomed and dressed, she reminds Aaron of the goddess Kali. She shouts angrily, "He's right!"

Sarah frowns and says peremptorily, "Sit down now, Siobhan. Parvati, remind us of the role of audience members."

Parvati says, "Before we speak, we take responsibility for transforming any sterile or hell states so as to speak from light rather than darkness. We—"

"She's the source of darkness!" the stunning beauty next to Siobhan declares. She jumps up and points an accusing finger at the actress, and twists the bright red lei that she is wearing.

Aaron feels Sarah working very hard to transform her own state and the states of all those affected by Leilani's outburst. Yukie intensifies her fertile state until it joins and strengthens that of the group. After a pause, Sarah replies kindly, "Good heavens, Leilani, you know that the actress is improvising and is in character."

"She shouldn't shout at Aaron!"

"You have two choices. You can leave now, or recover a fertile state and speak when you're ready."

Leilani sits. Her expression goes blank, but Aaron can feel the sisters' rage interfering with the fertile state of the audience.

When the sisters remain silent, Sarah prompts, "Go on, Parvati."

"We use rules developed by Quakers for their unprogrammed meetings. We speak only when the spirit moves us, and only in a state of loving accord."

A fertility guilder stands and asks Connie kindly, "Why are you so angry?"

Connie's mouth closes and twists. She replies in a high, tense voice, "Don't be nice to me! You'll make me cry, and I'll lose all credibility in this boy's club. They can't abide any female who acts like a mother."

"Is that why you're angry?"

"I'm angry because I'm paid to do the wrong thing!"

"What do you mean?"

"They should send me here to find out what's wrong and why and how to fix it. Instead, they send me here to pretend we've got everything under control and to sweep every clue under the rug. They're terrified of the public, and always resort to bombast and bamboozling. They betray the patients, which means that I have to do that too. I hate this job!"

"That isn't fair," John says. "The job has a political dimension, and you knew that when you took it."

The actress looks pleadingly at Sarah, who says, "Björn? Can you cut the radio and television messages? I didn't realize how irritating they'd be! I think we made our point!"

The sound goes off, and the theater becomes silent. As the audience realizes its relief, scattered applause rises and spreads throughout the theater. The birds gradually resume singing. Aaron relaxes as the dark fixations fed by media lift.

Sarah laughs with relief and continues, "Thank you, Björn! We can learn a lot from that alone. Before we talk about what to learn from the enactment, let's take a few minutes to acknowledge that our species created enormous peril, and that we will be working all our lives to remedy it." As the audience focuses, she adds, "Now let's contemplate and appreciate the work that each of us has done to restore the body of life to health … and the work that we are doing now … and the work that we will do in the future."

After several minutes, Yukie says, "I let my focus narrow

to the foreground. I didn't see Connie's or Melissa's perceptual errors."

Sarah says, "Thanks for that. Anyone else?"

A woman wearing the pocket-studded field pants of the restoration guild stands and says, "Their expectations were formed by the habits acquired by the body of humanity. I try to allow the bodies of habitats and life to shape my entrained states through my core, but my focus narrowed, too, which must mean that I hold modern habits."

"How many of you found that your focus narrowed?"

A large percentage of people raise their hands.

"How many think the noise narrowed it?"

As many hands go up, another restoration guilder stands and says, "My focus didn't narrow. I've just come from a remote restoration site where my senses were long attuned to habitat. Life in the nucleated village may be the cause of narrowing. Our core energies may diffuse. We might do better living in scattered tree houses and gathering once a week."

Sarah gasps. "That's a big one! We'll have to hold that possibility for a long time—years perhaps. Good. Anything else?"

A fabro guilder stands and says, "In soft fabro, we're together all day and we focus the way Connie and Melissa do. That can be a good thing—if we use it to purify and intensify interbeing."

An agro guilder in the denim coveralls of his guild rises and says, "We may need a psychosocial guild."

A trader wearing the all-weather tricorn guild hat adds, "Or a guild of guilds to hold the others."

One of the schoolers pipes up, "Sarah's our social guild."

Sarah laughs. "That would be a problem, wouldn't it? No one can do that work for others; I do it with all of you. Any other weighty questions to hold?"

Aaron says, "I've been noticing the time credits they're form-ing. They're seeing and connecting with a larger view of life that will lead to our view of the body of life and to the role of our species as the immune system of the body of life and—"

"Stop for a moment. John?"

"I agree," John says. "We were beginning to practice as we do now, but we didn't have the perspective to see that."

Sarah nods to Aaron, who continues, "They're also creating cure states that join being with doing. Judging by the state of the actress, I would guess that Mom was almost always in a cure state at that time, and that her egalitarian, sororal love of Pea helped to form the care state in which she later held her cure states, and that led to her way of joining being and doing."

"So," Sarah says thoughtfully, "they were joining being and doing and context. That is huge, isn't it?"

Onstage, the actress playing Melissa says, "Ahem!"

Sarah, John, and Aaron turn in surprise and then look at each other and smile. Sarah laughs, and says, "That's just what Melissa would have done!"

Yukie says hastily, "Go!"

A few scenes later, several members of the audience, including the beautiful sisters, clash like metal against the cymbals of their known history. In the enactment's action, Pea—then known as Connie rather than either Consuela or Pea—visits a priest in the hospital. Aaron has learned—to his surprise—that Connie's birth father was a priest, and that the kindly old friend of the family known as Father Sean had stepped up to father Connie and to grandfather Rose.

The set is a hospital room, and Connie is standing by Father

Sean's bedside. He has been admitted for a possible heart attack. Connie says, "You can go home today if your tests are negative. If so, may I visit you tomorrow at your rectory?"

"You'll be as welcome as the dawn," he says, patting her hand kindly. "But there is something I should tell you now, in case … well, in case of in case." When they have spoken of her father, the lights go down.

A voice says, "I see a time credit here. He is about to father her."

Sarah says, "Stop! Lights please."

The lights come up. A fertility guilder stands and says, "I believe that this is the first instance of child sharing in our lineal history. That makes it the first step in our adoption of the Hawaiian kinship structure in which older generations raise younger ones. That allows us to treat the community as a kindred, to dissociate fertility from childbearing, and to express sexuality fully and freely—and ethically and stably."

Sarah smiles. "Put that way, it's a tremendous time credit!"

A restoration guilder stands and says, "It's bigger than that! Child sharing allowed us to decrease our numbers rapidly, and to ease the pressure that our teaching puts on this habitat. Had we not found a way to decrease our numbers, we might have multiplied and been party to threatening the last 300 million years of growth and development of the body of life."

A schooler stands and says, "It's even bigger. Our family makes it possible for kids to take the initiative in their own development. We can choose mentors, and develop creativity however we're able as soon as we're able."

Sarah says in amazement, "Well done, you three! You reframed our time credits in a way that recognizes Consuela Martín's contribution and integrates our kindred's lifework!"

The audience applauds.

A restoration guilder sitting on a cycle in the far back, just inside the ring of alders, stands. As Sarah gestures for quiet, and the applause dies out, the restoration guilder says, "I just want to add that without this moment in our lineage, we might have focused on DNA and genetics and lost sight of the fullness of the body and the central importance of transmitting being and doing."

Leilani stands abruptly and extends her hand high above her head.

Sarah nods to her.

Leilani begins calmly, but ends in an anguished outburst. "You talk as if you could transmit a being apart from blood. Pea's being belongs to us, not to Aaron! He was nothing to my family!"

The audience gasps.

John replies kindly, "Pea wouldn't have seen it that way, Leilani. She was acutely aware of her short stature. She made a point of distinguishing the unusual from the abnormal. She used social Darwinism, eugenics, and Nazi idolatry of the übermensch to illustrate late modern misperceptions of about genetics, and to show that humans can't tell adaptive traits from maladaptive ones."

Parvati says, "When I researched Connie's life, I discovered that she had been talking with Melissa when she recognized that we can't manage what we don't understand, and that we understand too little of the body of life to manage it. She hoped that we could learn to work with it, and helped Reggie form the view that our species might take the role of neuroimmunity in the body of life. We attributed it to Melissa, but Connie was present for the realization."

"Before you get too cozy, I just want to point out that all humans have genes—and blood—and that this kindred isn't the only one to come to the same conclusions."

"Good grounding, Doug," Sarah says.

"If all of this is true," Leilani objects, "why did she encourage our mother to become a geneticist?"

"It was a good career move," Doug replies. "Pea was always worried about money and she—and all of us—let money do our thinking. Money made some godawful decisions—and some good ones."

John says, "Genetics continue to be important at the level of mechanism. As Pea liked to point out, poisons harm everyone, and genes determine how they harm each individual—whether it's dementia or cancer or chronic poisoning or something else. But genes don't do that alone, they do it with epigenetic factors, diet, and myriads of other factors. Genes play an important role, and genetic testing continues to inform us, but testing can also easily lead us astray. Like any kind of molecularism, it fixates our attention on minutia and distracts us from the human scale, and from definitive care and cure."

Aaron adds, "Pea used to focus on the environment, and how changing conditions can turn a helpful gene into a harmful one, and vice versa."

"What? Tell me how!" Leilani demands truculently. "Give me an example!"

John says, "Sickle cell anemia. People with two copies of the gene have crises in which small areas of tissue die. Over time, they may lose whole organs. The gene persists because people with one copy are less susceptible to malaria."

Aaron adds kindly, "I just want to say that when I knew

Connie, she was the sweetest and most loving of all my mother's friends, and I called her Auntie."

Leilani looks at him skeptically. Gradually, her expression shifts to wonder and then desire. Yukie's heart sinks. She has seen this before: Leilani wants to breed with Aaron. Aaron overhears as she whispers to Rafa, "Your uncle had better watch out for her. I think she wants to breed with him."

To Yukie's relief, Sarah says, "Thank you everyone. Go!"

Toward the end, when Aaron is overtaxed by new and jarring information and overstimulated by the intense engagement of the audience, the enactment is reframed by the Melissa character saying, "I can see that we were born in a special time, and are the only ones who can put our house in order before it's too late."

The stage lights go down.

Yukie says, "I struggle to forgive the ancestors, and this shows that their problems began long before they were born—like ours did."

After applauding the performers, Aaron excuses himself as soon as he deems polite—or perhaps a little sooner. He heads west hundreds of yards to stand on a rocky outcropping, seeing as far as he can see out over Cowichan Bay and its environs to the hills on the horizon. He is remembering things now that he has not thought of since childhood, and feels as if invisible strings have run through him and are pulling bits of his embodied experience from one place to the other. How little and how much he absorbed as a child! How the tensions of that time continue to impel him forward, and how easing them removes the obstacles in his way! He is carried away by a rising memory of the shock of his first visit here, when he stood on this very rock. Sitting down, he lets memory and order run wild. After some hours, he realizes that his breath is easing and that he is hungry.

Aaron retraces his steps down the path to the lodge, ready to see his family's past through the eyes of this community. Two things have fallen into place in his mind already. One is that Pea's legacy is an example of how one conscientious person can become like a catherine wheel that sends out blessings in all directions, and how any one of those blessings—harsh or sweet—can catalyze transformation. Another is that the actress playing his mother when she was young and confident and healthy has captured his imagination. Seeing her in this ghostly way is both breaking and filling his heart. He hopes that seeing her legacy will help him to put her to rest and also to sustain her memory.

2
Melissa's Legacy

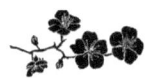

A week later, after Aaron and Parvati have talked through the first enactment, Parvati listens as Sarah welcomes the audience to the second one. The black and white image of the friendship group on the day they met in 1972, which shows them in the common room of their college dormitory, is displayed on the central panel. Then the stage lights come up on the set that recreates that room, and on the actors who will be playing the friendship group. The latter are seated just like their counterparts in the photo. Sarah asks John to introduce the friends.

Looking on, Parvati is stunned. Sarah gave fair warning that she would improvise more this time, but Parvati didn't expect Sarah to cut the photo montage that they had so carefully and laboriously prepared, or to leave out the introductory remarks that they had crafted to convey the conditions of the time.

Parvati feels suddenly stripped bare, all too aware of having taken Aaron's life in her hands and of having done with it something that she has never done and does not know how to do. She fears that he will dislike it, or worse—that she will make a mistake, or divide him from his legacy, or discourage him. She puts anxious thoughts aside to focus on Sarah, who seems to have taken for granted that the audience knows the era of her youth. Parvati must find a way to convey it to them in a few sentences.

She must think fast.

John introduces the actor who will be playing the young Doug, who is sprawled in an easy chair and who—with his sideburns and fake freckles—closely resembles the original. John explains that the young Doug was a big man and very bright, and learned to act like a clown to avoid intimidating people. The old Doug objects, and gets a laugh. John then introduces the young Sarah as a blonde bombshell who was preparing for her role as personal dramatist for an entire community. The old Sarah turns up her hands and gets a laugh.

Parvati's mind races back over the events of the time. She pictures Melissa and Pea feeling uneasy, and Melissa and John—along with the whole of the species—trying stances of mutual care of the kind that led to breakthroughs like international law, peaceful social change, and the eradication of smallpox. They were discerning problems and solutions that would begin to reveal the destined role of humans in the body of life.

John introduces April as a prim farm girl; Alan as a Jewish boy who had never left Brooklyn; himself as a skinny kid from the northwoods who played the music of older men and had never kissed a girl; and Melissa as a sober scholar with a round face, bug-eyed glasses, and wholesome outlook that concealed an old soul. John then introduces Randall as a California boy who was even more attractive to women than the actor, and who had experimented with love-ins and encounter sessions. Parvati is surprised and touched by the undying jealousy in John's tone. Lastly, he introduces Zeke as the smartest of the set.

A set of older actors enters. Each takes a place behind a younger actor, and Sarah introduces them as the ones who will play the friends in middle age. Parvati sees life in time folding in on itself. Her mind clears. It is as if she, too, were Melissa and John, and could wheel away the backboards and reveal the hidden sources of human actions—including errors that they wanted to conceal, and perennial habits of narrow denial, or diffuse focus, disregard or post-hoc rationalization.

Parvati begins to speak, trusting her train of thought to reach its destination. "Last week, in the saga of Melissa and Pea, we saw our antecedents at a time in human history when they became aware that they were missing something of critical importance. This week, we will see Melissa and John grapple with human limitations, recognize the horrific errors of their time, and attempt to right those errors in their own lives. We will also see them stop short of creating the solutions that will be realized in the next enactment."

Parvati hears a man on stage clear his throat deliberately. The real Sarah laughs, and says, "Let's not forgot Professor Weitzman and his wife! The professor was a Jewish refugee from Nazi Germany who had a classical European education and who served as resident master of our dormitory. His wife was also a refugee."

A light rain begins to patter on the membrane roof that Björn put up at dawn. A chill wind whooshes through the theater.

Parvati is glad that she spread word yesterday that Sarah may propose that Melissa and John be declared founders. The seats are filled today, and even Leilani and Siobhan are taking in the story rather than reacting before thinking. While Melissa's work is known here, few know of her life and even fewer of her and John's life work on the science of everyday life. Parvati looks for Björn, and nods to him. As the lights go down, she glances carefully at Aaron, who smiles.

Sarah expects this day to be much more difficult for Aaron,

as his mother had spoken little of the college years that formed their friendship group. Parvati had hesitated to include those years in the enactment, but there was no other way to convey the soul bond between Melissa and John that the community might count as a full consortship, or—as Sarah intends to argue—as a partial one. The community has not recognized partial consortships, nor considered them as fertile couplings that might give birth to a third. To view their own community as having in part arisen from such a bond will stretch their world view and—Sarah hopes—revive their creativity and spur its evolution. Fortunately, Parvati's entanglement with Aaron is already so multifaceted and intense that she should be able to hold him if he becomes upset, and to help him reconcile with it afterward.

The lights come up on the young characters on their first day at the University of Chicago in the early 1970s. As the resident master welcomes them and tells them of the dangers of the inner city, images of the assassination of Dr. King, of the riots and destruction of vast stretches of the surrounding neighborhood, and of gangs and prisons and rapes and murders and drug use appear on the screen. Parvati can feel revulsion rising in the community and sorrow welling up in Aaron. This history is familiar to him.

As the scenes of freshman year go by, Aaron and the community are shocked to witness Sarah and Doug fall into an unstable pattern of approach and avoidance darkened by cycles of aggression and pain; delighted by John's musical skills; mystified by the egg-head education that seems little different than that endured by medieval scribes; and amused by the failure of John and Melissa to recognize the bond forming between them. The audience and Aaron are entranced when John goes off to old

Alaska to work in an aging cannery, passing close by Saltspring Island when traveling back and forth on the ferry that to this day follows a course along the inside passage. They are shocked, though, when Melissa, dismayed at being the only virgin, and Randall, dismayed at being left out of the inner circle of intellectuals, have a summer affair. Parvati has to freeze the action onstage while the audience, unable to reconcile with this knowledge in silence, breaks into personal conversations that rise, spread, and eventually die out. At first, she feels nothing from Aaron, but as the action continues, she realizes that he is in shock. The nature of his mother's bond with Randall was unknown to him; it is also one that Sarah will be proposing as a partial consortship.

As Aaron becomes more and more upset, Parvati shares his state and transforms it. She had not expected this to be a problem and acknowledges her regret by taking his hand and clasping it, palm to palm. He squeezes her hand, and his eyes search her face. He is puzzled and wary. She whispers, "I didn't realize that this would upset you. Shall I stop the action?"

He whispers back, "I'd like an intermission after this scene. Ten minutes, or longer."

At the end of the scene, Parvati calls for half an hour's break and suggests that each attendee take time to process any unexpected revelation. She looks at Sarah, who introduces the topic of partial consortship and announces the chance for personal discussion during the interval, and for community discussion after the enactment in the forest sanctuary, to be led by the elders of the fertility guild.

As Aaron gets up to leave, Parvati asks, "May I join you?"

Aaron reaches out to help her up. She can see that his trust in her is shaken, and may be broken. She will repair it if she can, with trust and transparency. She follows him up the trail that leads toward concepto, restoro, and the memorial. "There is a stump in the woods to the right, if you'd like a private place to sit."

He stops and follows her off the trail. Sitting on a fallen log, she waits patiently to know his thoughts. Aaron sighs and seats himself on the stump. "It seems that Sarah is using my family's past to make some changes; I didn't expect that. And I didn't expect such a personal revelation. Mom seems to have gotten around back then."

He is holding back. She says, "Your legacy is part of our community. Your mother is one of the mothers of our community. The others had consorts and with them took this community as their third. Their role was obvious. We are only now becoming aware that although she had no consort as we know it, and had children and a grandchild, we are—as best we can tell—a third to her. We are beginning—with your legacy—to integrate her true role into our narrative."

"What is this third? It makes no sense to me."

"When two people come together in union—especially a sexual union—something new comes into being. This is how we define fertility. If it persists and takes a life-giving or generative—that is, reproductive—form, we consider it a child. It may be a spirit child, or a brain child, or a baby."

"So in your view, my mother is your mother."

"Yes, exactly," Parvati affirms.

"I'm not jealous. This isn't like finding out that she had other children before us. This is like finding out that I'm your brother. I don't—I can't get my head around it."

"In India, we have what's called the guru in large form, which is a bit like the body of Christ, or the body of life. When the guru dies and the followers gather, we see them as the living body of the guru."

"No offense, but that doesn't help."

"Think of Old America's founding fathers, then."

"So ... Mom was a founding mother."

"Yes, of this community—and perhaps of individuals whose lives were changed by her."

"So ... you want me to be a founding son?"

"I hadn't thought of it that way. I would say that I want you to be one of the elders who evolves our starting premises—many of which we now know came from your mother."

"You have plenty of elders."

"True, but most of them were taught by the people we already recognize as founders. We believe that you were taught by her and may be able to return her teachings to us."

"Tell me now: Will we be seeing her with John, too?"

"Yes."

"That will be like having more than one father. Like having three," John says. "Can you tell how Rafa is taking this?" he asks gently.

Parvarti is non-plussed. She never considered that point of view. "I believe that she's curious, and perhaps better able to understand her grandmother."

Aaron ponders for a moment and asks, "Can I sit this one out?"

"We can delay it, but many people have come a long way to see it."

"What do you think we should do?"

"I think we should face her life, and that you should let me and the others support you as you encounter it as she did—or as nearly as we can present it."

"Isn't that union?"

Parvati smiles. "Yes, of the kind that we practice as a group. We call it the group mind, or shared interbeing."

Aaron stands up and grunts. "This is a lot at once."

"If we focus on her story now, and take as much time as we need to put it into our context and yours, and to integrate it into our thinking, it will be easier for you to do the inner work of reconciling your narrative of her with what we know of her life and its impact on us."

Aaron sighs and reaches out his hand; rising, she takes it. He says ruefully, "I'm going to have to lean on you, and I'm going to be heavy!"

She puts her other hand over his and says, "I'm sorry. I didn't foresee this. Can you tell me why this is so difficult?"

"My story of her is of a sexually and religiously conservative woman who fit in very well in the Amanas—with the exception of her Judaism. I thought she and Dad had problems because she didn't want sex."

Paravarti shakes her head and then says, "Shall I tell you one more thing?"

"Go ahead, shoot."

"She never converted. Not formally."

Aaron sighs with relief. "That much I know. Dad—who was born Jewish—didn't like religion, but he agreed to let us have bar mitzvahs, and didn't stop her study or practice."

Later, as the lights go up again in the theater, Parvati feels Aaron surrender his separation and allow her full support to lift him. He is ready, now, to attend to this hidden story of college life and the life of the neighborhood around it, and for the tragic clash of the two that led to April's rape and brought his mother and

John together for several years, before ambition caused John to divide his life from hers. Aaron feels compassion and unexpected connection when John begins to weep quietly behind them.

When the next scene leaps ahead twenty years to a reunion of the two couples—John and Melissa, and Sarah and Doug—after Melissa has become ill, Aaron begins to smile, and to recognize background images from time to time. Like the audience, he is all attention when the actress playing Sarah tells her story of disenchantment with her job in D.C., and reacts when Jerome Junior appears and tells the story of his remodel of his father's restaurant. Only when Aaron hears clapping in a section of the theater does he look over and spot the elderly Jerome Junior and realize that the man's son, Jerome Beaulieu III, nicknamed Jerbeau, is playing his own grandfather.

Aaron feels a frisson as time telescopes three generations, spanning the end of modernity and the emergence of the age of life in time. His mother is at first the same age as her granddaughter, and her century-old friends watch their younger selves at the beginning and middle of their adult lives. When the middle-aged Sarah outs his mother's illness, he feels a bootless urge to rewind time to the point before she entered into a shell of pain and suffering. He barely listens as the fertility guilders point out the friends' errors of omission and commission, and then dispute how to detect their own now.

A voice says in the darkness, "I propose that we offer a drumming out after this enactment." The lights go up. A hospitality guilder stands in the center of the rows of folding seats that have been placed where the thrust stage was last time. "We're taking in far more old time debts this time."

Sarah says, "Yes, and we've reconciled or are reconciling

some of them, but most of the errors of mind that we've seen are still with us."

Parvati says, "We continue to take our happiness for granted, to imagine that we're separate from others, to define phenomena as if that alone managed our reality. We still attempt to control others or to act in their place; to get ahead of them as if they didn't belong to the same body of life; to avoid pain in others by assuming that it isn't our business, or our fault, or our fate. And I have no way to teach the schoolers to do better—except to slow things down, nurture perceptiveness and responsibility, and encourage them to look for and remedy their own errors."

A fertility guilder stands and says, "We're working on a way to teach children to become aware of cognitive errors, and to set them aside so as to strengthen entrained stances for restoration. Now that we've met Aaron, we're considering how to use care states. That may keep us busy for years. I don't see how we can do more."

Sarah says, "Our strengths lie in fertility and restoration, and all of our present guilds are catalyzing the recovery of the body of life. That's our mission. But we haven't learned to see beyond what we already know."

John says, "Think of it in terms of calculus. You've achieved velocity and momentum but your first and higher derivatives remain constants."

Belatanu stands and adds impatiently, "We're doing more than we can or should already. You're asking us to do more. You're trying to create a Utopia."

Dirk stands and points out, "It isn't a question of doing, it's a question of states of being. We don't want to get distracted by modern ideas of productivity or efficiency—or nihilism—or by older habits of fatalism. If we look ahead to a time in the near future when our states are stronger, our cores are more open and unbounded, and our awareness is permeating our bodies and beings and extending farther into the body of life, we will be better able to avoid being tools of our errors—including the error of confusing being and doing. " He continues, "Stances help too. Our radical reduction of malicious states is making it easier to hold intense fertile states that help us to outmaneuver malefactors."

An older warrior sitting beside Dirk stands in the center section, puts her hand on her heart, and says, "If we focus too narrowly, and view errors as irrelevant, we may overlook those that propel our growth and development and evolution. We may erase the ones that could lead us to our future."

Aaron squeezes Parvati's hand and says to those who have stood up, "I think I see one of the problems. You may be in sync with—or just ahead of—the moving front of time with respect to some guild processes, but not others. You may be moving forward unevenly."

Sarah laughs with delight and says, "Good. This is what the enactments are designed to do."

John says, "I just want to point out that in this enactment, the past, present, and unknown future are telescoped so that they reveal each other. This is revealing aspects of Melissa's life that I never understood. She's the main character of these enactments and is still living—in those who knew her, at least. But she's hidden, all but inaccessible. She isn't like an old tyrant, like Caesar, whose will and consequences you could see in the material world. She was a carer whose life was quiet and hidden and complex. The indirect consequences of her actions matter much more than the direct ones, which means that we can only meet her through those of us who knew her—or who were influenced by her."

Sarah says, "We hope that the enactments can help us to know Melissa as she was in time—in the time periods in which she lived, in her lifecycle, in lifecycles entangled with hers, and in life as a whole. In fact," Sarah adds dramatically, "we could see life in time as the main character of our enactments, and Melissa as the lens through which the founders were able to see the body of humanity and its accelerating erosion of the body of life."

Parvati is surprised when Doug chimes in, with uncharacteristic gravity, "The trick is to monitor errors that cause the body of humanity to lag behind or to move backward. If our little crew hadn't been so conformist, we might have seen possibilities other than going along or going against, and many extinct species might be alive today."

Sarah says, "I think we all agree that this community will not be doing more, or doing or redoing any particular thing. We can't change the past or present. We are changing the future, and we can become familiar enough with the past and present to act wisely in life, in time—in our present rather than past context—and so change the way we change the future."

Parvati says, "If we open our perceptions to what we don't see now but would want to see in a better future, we'll be able to create that future."

Belatanu sighs with exasperation. "Now you're talking time travel, and that's out of the question."

Parvati says kindly, "We are doing it now—in the form of a thought experiment."

Sarah says, "Let's take five minutes to look at something we don't want to see and consider the potential consequences of seeing it and acting differently."

The lights dim. After a time, a tiny bell rings offstage. The lights go up.

Léon stands and says, "I think I'm a man out of place, and Leilani's a woman out of time." Leilani is on her feet in a flash and about to retort when a child pulls her arm; she sits back down reluctantly. Léon continues, "That's a big revelation for me. I'll be thinking about it—and the hot and cold wars of the past century that took our species out of place and time."

Sarah says, "Thanks for that thought. What does the fertility guild think of it?"

One fertility guilder calls out, "I think we're overwhelmed. We can hold these ideas—but only if all of us share our strongest fertility states."

Another calls out, "We can't do that. Our energy bodies are entangled with place and time, and we're being asked to weaken that entanglement—or to imagine that we are. That will cost more energy than we can create."

"What does the warrior guild think?" Rafa asks Dirk.

"Modern errors disentangled us. Stances of malice are classic cases in point. They undo personal and interpersonal aggregation, and lineal continuity, and orientation to life in time. That creates and accelerates undoing. Luckily, we took the undoing of the last century as a chance to create new ways. But our work is still very perilous. We have to stay alert for fertile moments when the way forward opens without effort, and creation proceeds with ease."

Oke Ten stands and states, "This is one of those moments."

Parvati looks at Sarah, who is holding her breath. Oke Ten has been very reserved until now. He rarely follows where the young lead, but when he does, the older warriors join him.

Oke Ten goes on to say, "We are engaging thoughts that are new to us—or newly aggregated. If we focus and remain alert, we will be able to see new openings created by those errors that we do not drum out."

After a very long pause, during which the theater waits in silence, Sarah says in a warm tone of warning, "And then if we are not independent, free, and responsible we will turn to a teacher, founder, or elder and try copy them, or do what they tell us to do—or the opposite in Doug's case," she adds with a reluctant laugh. "Today, we will watch John and Melissa face the unknown and struggle to discover what no one knows and to do the right thing according to their lights. This is how we can found an evolving future."

Parvati says, "We're seeing John and Melissa face circumstances that made it difficult for them to avoid biological reality. Let's see if we can respond more nimbly to our reality. That will bring us closer to syncing, and to staying in sync!"

Sarah says, "Let's take five minutes to contemplate this dialogue."

The lights dim. When they go up again, Parvati declares boldly, "Now, let's return to the narrative and see what we can glean from it." The lights go down.

In the next scenes, they see Melissa—who is too sick to research the medical database or to keep many variables in her head—collaborate with John, who is now a professor, and with whom she can share and develop ideas as with no one else. Between her informed observations and his facility with identifying useful medical knowledge and designing experiments, they find the causes of her ailments.

Through this, they recognize that she and untold others are suffering from human-caused ailments, that human error has always caused ailments by undoing evolved systems, and that the natural antidotes and healthy habitats that could cure them were being inadvertently eradicated. They realize that the social response to Rachel Carson's *Silent Spring* made things much worse through the attempt to control hazards one at a time, which was like trying to empty the ocean with a teaspoon.

When the scene in which they make these discoveries ends, the audience stands and applauds. After a time of rejuvenating affirmation of the source of the solutions that they presently embody, they discuss—for the rest of the day, and for days and weeks to come—the possibility of updating their approach to the science of everyday life in order to better sync with time.

3

Coming of Age

That night, Belatanu leads Rafa out of the dining room and through the front door of the lodge toward the agro center. Rafa inhales the cooling mist and enjoys the moisture gathering on her skin and refreshing her spent flesh. She is quiet now, calm, aware of the profound pleasure of immersing her being in her companion's serene grounding. She feels safe with him; safe even from the shadow of death that never leaves her, and that she would like to elude.

They make their way across the uneven ground with high steps, pinlights out to avoid stepping in fresh manure, and enter through the massive, creaking barn door to take refuge in the warm, straw-strewn interior that Belatanu calls his nest. He goes to the sheep enclosure. A wooly flock gets up and approaches. Rafa enters the enclosure, pats them, and plops down on the straw. A sheep lies down in front of her, and she strokes its belly.

"You like animals?" Bel asks.

"I love wild ones. I've never met animals that I could get cozy with. I had no idea that sheep were so sweet!"

"They like the way we care for them—and they love being mothered like that."

"Why did you choose agro for vocation?" Rafa asks.

"I always loved it, and always took it for granted, even after

I got to know ducks and salmon. For a while, I was all set to be a trader or a forager. I love land and sea navigation—but then—believe it or not—I realized I was enjoying composting as part of soil production and knew it was what I had to do."

"Composting?"

"Manure and all. Precious stuff, that."

"I … I love our third."

"What?" he asks, with a note of disapproval.

"I feel something that comes from us. Don't you?"

"You don't know this place. We do things differently here. I'm still getting used to it, and I got here at fourteen."

"How old are you now?"

Belatanu grips the rail of the sheep enclosure and looks down. "Twenty-seven."

"Is that a problem?"

"It's old for never having had a consort."

"Did anyone initiate you—you know, sexually?"

Belatanu nods. Rafa looks at him. She senses unspoken words. Finally, he says, "I'm pretty sure it was Leilani."

"You don't know?"

"It's a rite in darkness. You're not supposed to know. But she has a scar on her back and piercings on her … body."

"Did you … enjoy it?"

"Hate, yeah."

"What do you want in a consort?"

"Someone who knows what they're doing?"

"These enactments are my initiation. Teach me."

He tells her of the manners, mores, and practices that Reggie and Graeme established to enhance the chances that each individual would find a consort with whom to become an abler soul—that is, more than the sum of their souls, and in some cases much, much more. Children begin to learn the sevenfold model of the body when they are under seven: awareness, understanding, perceptions, sensations, energy, flesh, and interbeing; they also learn to ground themselves in the energy centers of the body and in life and place and time. They practice group union of all but flesh, and learn to unite with family and community to further their preparation for adult life.

"I think that's universal," Rafa remarks. "But not usually as deliberate."

"Yes. I grew up with something like it. But the art of it is rare now in post-modern times, and rarely as complete and consensual and constructive."

"I think I can do that. Do you?"

"I don't know."

"Are you willing to try?" Rafa persists.

"I don't know."

"What are the other barriers?"

"Commitment."

"I'm good for a year. You?"

He nods.

"What else?"

"Birth control. I don't want a child as my third."

"Are you fertile?"

He nods. "We don't have the cut until we have become creative in our vocation, and have discerned our first third with a consort."

"I'm not. I had what you call the cut. And we're both simple-diffs. And Doug and Björn have approved my fabro trader project so that my proposal—and my time with Doug—count as my initiation project, and carrying it out will count as my vocation project."

"You haven't been initiated sexually."

"I'm experienced."

Belatanu's face falls. He feels unbearably sad to her. "Then you definitely need to be initiated. You'll have developed patterns that are ... not the best."

"You want me to have sex with a stranger who might not even be a stranger?"

"I want you to be patterned by someone who is gifted in the body."

"I don't know if I can do that. What else?"

"We drum out as many burdens as possible. And you and I have a lot—you more than I. I can feel them."

"How bad is it?"

"Bad."

"Is that why you don't want me?"

"That's why this will be very hard for you."

She notices that he says "will" and asks, "What do we have to do to be ready?"

"You should start your purification work and undergo sexual initiation. And then do drumming out every day until nothing more comes. We can do that together. And then, when you're ready, we can join."

"I may not get there." She tells him of her time on the streets, beginning as a neglected daughter who sought safety in a pack of friends and ending with her escape to the mountains. He first looks shocked and then sadder and sadder until—after she finishes—he bursts into tears. She wants to hug him and comfort him, but holds back. He has not given her permission. She sighs and lies down by a sheep, yawning. Belatanu shakes his head vigorously and draws her to her feet. He clears his throat. "Don't fall asleep! If we unite here at the dream level, which is unconscious, we may never be able to form a conscious union."

"What if I'm never ready?"

"You will be. You'll see when we do the drumming out. We can start tomorrow morning, when we're fresh."

A week later, Rafa waits anxiously on the stack of futons that rests on top of a tatami mat. A masked fertility guilder retrieved her from the purification ritual at midnight and led her in silence to a private refuge in the woods behind the fertility center, where she bathed in rosemary and juniper berry oils, and lay in a warming box as scented warm oil drizzled down on her third eye. She entered an altered state that was more refreshing than sleep. Then, after some time—she knows not how long—the masked guilder led her to this room, had her lie on the futons, covered her with a towel, and turned out the room and hall lights. She can see nothing, expect nothing, control nothing. She can only trust to sacred life and love and the knowledge of the body kept in this mysterious—to her—place.

Some time later, the door opens and closes, and someone circles the futons. Rafa feels anxious. She is not sure where the person is, which makes it seem as if the person is everywhere. After a time, she senses someone near her head and feels a hand brush her forehead with exquisite tenderness; then gentle hands cradle the back of her head. Vivid images of the Rocky Mountains seem forced out of Rafa's memory into her present view. She frowns. Her visual field goes dark but for diffuse blue light. The hands move to her crown; once again, she goes into a state that is more restful than sleep and does not stir as, Reiki-like, the hands give and take energy at many points on her covered body. Then, the door opens and closes again, leaving her alone. It was a reading of some kind, perhaps, by a sensitive who is not an initiator. She wants to understand, but would rather sleep.

Rafa hears the door once more, and someone slips in to lie beside her. She is at first uncomfortably aware of the person, then dozes again and becomes used to the presence, which is gentle and loving. Arms lift her to a sitting position. The person—the initiator, it seems—sits opposite and touches foreheads, arms, and legs. Rafa cannot tell anything about the person's flesh, and is unexpectedly unconcerned as she feels the initiator's intangible body merge with hers. When the merging is complete, Rafa feels no third, and no otherness. The initiator is like a mirror who has become an extension of Rafa. She is almost surprised to hear the initiator draw breath, and then feels a state of arousal that belongs to her and to her larger self. The initiator stops before her arousal intensifies. Rafa realizes that the initiator is repatterning her.

It is a kind of sexual intrusion that she attempts to accept freely by picturing Belatanu. Her arousal abruptly escalates: it is a simulation, a mediation; not an intrusion. The initiator is absent as an individual. The initiator inhales sharply and then withdraws with a delicate caress of her crown, leaving Rafa suddenly sad. She does not know if the union went well or went wrong; she guesses that she has disrupted the process by intruding on the initiator. It is all so alien to her. She lies down, deflated by the anticlimax. She is not sure what to do. This is more difficult than she expected, and in a different way. If the initiator returns, she must find a way to feel that she is joining with Belatanu through the initiator.

The door opens and closes again. Rafa waits. It is her intention to surrender to, and to cooperate with, this experience that Belatanu believes essential. She does not want to let him down, or to mar their enjoyment of each other. If nothing else, it will put his mind at rest and obviate compunctions that she may never understand. Again, arms lift her. The energy is different; she is fairly certain this is someone else. The anonymity is unnerving, but if it were Yukie or Björn, she would not want to know. Again, they touch foreheads and merge as if the initiator is Bel; they become one body and being. This transports her. She clearly visualizes Belatanu's eyes, into which she has been gazing daily.

This time, the illusion that she is with him is complete, and she feels aroused in the way she does when she is near him and mad for him. Now the process flows like a clear and quiet stream. She responds and is adjusted and adjusted again until her whole body—and every hair on her skin—reaches a bliss of union. She is flooded by blinding, searing light that joins the living bodies entangled with her and her consort. It is like rising beyond the surface of a sea of profane confusion. She is one with all that they are, and the physical initiation has yet to begin.

Rafa stops on the trail to look up. She can't see or hear anything. She scans the forest with her pinlight and spots a rope stair. She says quietly, "Léon?"

"Back here, on Siobhan's deck," comes a murmured reply.

Rafa listens closely. A hundred human voices murmur like birds in the canopy above. She says, "Do you want to come with Doug and me?"

"Anything but another night in the hammock!"

Rafa hears low laughter, quick footfalls, and a ripping sound.

She forms a mental picture of Léon hurrying across the deck and sliding down the stair rope. She becomes aware that she is cold in her shaven scalp and thin bark cloth, and that her adult initiation tattoo hurts. She places her palms on her scalp to hold in its warmth. In going from the sexual initiation rite to the last of the fabro initiation rite, she will be going from ecstasy to material want in the space of a day.

Léon's feet hit the ground with a blunt thud. "Live large!"

Voices high above murmur, "Love long!"

"Hey Rafa," calls a teasing voice that she recognizes as Belatanu's. "I hear you want to be a woman of the sea."

"If I have to pick a habitat, I pick that one."

Somber laughter spills over the deck rail. Belatanu coaxes Rafa, saying, "You don't like our fields? Our Cascadian forest?"

"I like the trails and the trade routes that take me places. That's why I want to be a fabro trader!"

"Oh! You might have to choose the built environment," he says in the tone that he uses when he winks.

"Is that a habitat?"

"Is your nose on your face?"

"At this point, I'd have to check. Maybe it's yours."

After a beat, a murmur of knowing laughter spreads all the way to Léon, and they continue on the trail.

A beam of light lurches up the trail behind Rafa and Léon and sweeps back and forth, blinding Rafa and scattering sharp silhouettes across layers of boughs and tree trunks. Doug's shrunken silhouette passes them and thrashes ahead. Rafa smells the stench of alcohol. Doug is drunk.

Léon says to Doug, "The rite bans all lights before dawn."

"Fuck the rite!"

Rafa says uneasily, "I invited Léon."

Doug growls like a bear. Rafa and Léon rush to catch up. She realizes as they stumble along the trail that she may be tested by more than the purification ordeal. She wonders if his drunkenness is by design or by chance. She says kindly to Doug, "We all need quiet, and sleep."

"You sleep," Doug growls. "At my age you're never asleep and never awake—and finally you never wake up again—like Missy, damn her hide! I thought I could count on her!"

"*Tío's* taking her place."

Doug snorts, "Good thing. Your dad is like his dad. The ungrateful little shit didn't even visit."

Rafa says evenly, "I'm not him."

"Look, kid, Sarah wants us to say everything was for the best, but it wasn't. Your grandma and I struggled and fucked up and hung on by our fingernails, and I plan to remember her as she was until I'm in the ground."

Rafa inhales the breath of the fecund forest and replies gently, "Sarah and the rest are doing their grief work and reconciling their time debts."

"I'll give you that, kid," Doug allows. "They make the past serve the future—and I come here to enjoy the way they do it! But they want to make it look like Missy planned all this. They want to steal her life and her memory."

Rafa pauses and turns to whisper to Léon, "Do you want to go back?"

"Not yet. I want to hear this."

Doug stops, turns around, shines his light on Rafa and Léon and attacks. "Kids here live in a bubble. They can't handle outsiders and couldn't have handled the founders! Randall could be a pain in the ass—and so could your grandma. I won't let Sarah forget it! And you know what? That's why she invites me!"

"Tell us about Grandma. We want to know the truth."

"His truth," Léon mutters.

Doug turns and continues down the trail. After a few paces he asks testily, "Did you ask your uncle?"

"He said she didn't love Grandpa the way she should."

Doug grunts angrily. "I know what's going on here! Your dad treats your mom like a doormat and she takes it and you think she should. She shouldn't. And your grandma was worse. When she got sick your grandpa punished her and she helped. They shared nothing but blame and shame. It was the worst marriage I've ever seen, including mine—which was a money match. I've never loved like—" Doug's voice stops.

The three walk in a wordless line. Their steps raise smells of must and decay that blend with scents of evergreen from above. Rafa watches the light dance and memorizes the puddles, roots, and rocks ahead that are partly obscured by Doug's bony back. Rafa's heart contracts around her grandma's lost dreams and disappointed hopes and feels an urge to tell Doug that the old have no right to crush the hopes and dreams of the young. But Doug knows this already; he has been giving his all to her and to *Tío*, and is grieving for her grandma and spewing it out as rage. Rafa will try to follow the example of her peers and accept and reconcile sorrow. She will not respond in kind.

Ahead, the trail narrows and ducks left between a slick rock wall and an old growth snag. Rafa glimpses moss and ferns and seedlings atop the snag. Insects and birds have stripped away the bark, and fungi are flaking the remaining phloem. When she reaches the narrow place, she puts her hands out to the side to feel her way between wet rock and hollow bark.

Doug is breathing deeply and quickly, and soon attacks from a different and more difficult angle. "You had a grandma like no other. You should build her a monument. Your grandpa and dad were too mean and bitter to honor her memory and you never bothered to visit. You never even asked me about her when I visited you. Nothing hurt her as much as that—not even those decades of constant pain!"

Rafa feels the pull of Doug's sticky remorse. Her father has always taken his remorse out on others and she knows how to deflect it. But now, in the wee hours, after a night of ordeal and in the presence of a witness, she cannot escape her careless culpability. "I made an error of omission. We all make errors like that every day."

Doug sighs heavily and says guiltily. "She was trapped. I had plenty of cash. I had houses! I could have invited her to stay, given her a place to go. Christ! I could have funded her research. I had the social capital to get the word out, to change the course of history. But I knew she didn't care about my money and I wanted to keep it that way. It was stupid!"

"We all miss things. You can't change what happened. And why would you? Look at this place, and Grandma's and John's clinics. Everything did turn out for the best, like Sarah said."

Doug contradicts her in a mollified tone. "You have to see it that way, kid. Our actions created your givens."

Léon says kindly, "You do so much for us. We're all grateful. We're glad that you remember the founders and that we can remember them with you."

Doug walks twenty yards in silence. His mood turns maudlin. He is almost in tears as he says, "You're good kids, you know—the best."

Rafa follows Doug out of the dense boundary of the forest onto a paved road. When Léon emerges, the three turn right toward town. As they walk, Doug turns philosophical. "Part of Melissa lives on here, but not all of her. To love her was to know her. It wasn't easy. She could put you off. She could be bristly and picky and passionate about things that didn't seem to mean anything. But she was as deep as the river of life," he says, choking back tears. "She saw depths, and showed them to you."

At the main street of town, they turn toward the dark expanse of the harbor. Rafa smells low tide, the frames of the mussel farm north of the harbor, and seaweed and fish carcasses drying on racks. The gulls are sleeping and the onshore breeze has yet to rise. The sound of waves is muted by mist that blurs the pale moonlight revealing rooftops and deep-water dock.

"I didn't really feel her loss until now," Rafa says quietly.

Doug chokes back tears. "I see her in you kid, I really do. I was just—pissed, and pissed off."

The sound of their footsteps echoes against narrow blocks of townhomes, the doctor's office that stands on stilts above the produce market, and the care house where the disabled and elderly of the island sleep beneath a rooftop deck that overlooks the sea. Doug switches off his light. As their eyes adjust, Rafa sees pinpoint solar lights in the brickwork of the walkway. When they step out on a dock, their hollow steps jangle against the plashing waves and the creaking lines of boats moored along the shore.

Léon says tentatively, "Why didn't you and Sarah become consorts?"

"I was married and she had too many opinions."

"What about all those women you talk about?"

"You have no idea what it's like in the poison barrens. I take promising young women to a place where they won't be beaten or raped or brainwashed. I leave them better off and some choose to show their gratitude."

"Tell me more about Grandma," Rafa says.

Doug stops beside his boat and inhales deeply. "She was fiercely dedicated to right living. John wanted to make an impact, Sarah wanted to set the world to rights, I wanted strategic influence, but she wanted love and harmony for all. That's why John loved her—and why Randall did, too."

Doug clambers into the boat. Rafa unties the forward line; Léon unties the aft. She hops in and wraps the lines around the cleats. Léon remains on the dock. Doug turns on the strips of tiny blue lights that outline the boat and disappears below decks.

Léon says, "I think I'll go back."

"Was this too much?"

"Enough."

Doug reappears with glasses and a bottle that clink dully as he holds them up. "Best scotch in the world. Want a shot?"

"No, thanks," Léon says as he backs away.

As Léon disappears into the night, Rafa is glad. She thinks that her friend made a good choice, and she would leave too, if she were free of responsibilities. "Love life or leave it," she says bracingly.

"Be strong or be wrong," Léon replies, his voice sounding as near and as far as her grandma.

Doug goes to the helm and puts his bottle and glasses in a niche near the wheel. He takes command as if he has never left the boat. "Here's what happens next. First I'm going to have another drink, and then I'm going to sail you to a sheltered cove of Pender

Island, and then I'm going to put you in a dinghy. You'll lie in it and contemplate death until I pick you up."

"Will I have food or water?"

"They're in a box under the seat of the dinghy."

"What if it rains?"

"You'll know it when you feel it."

Doug pours a shot, downs it, and doubles over in a fit of coughing. When he recovers, he fills another glass and drops it over the edge into the sea. He says bracingly, "Here's to you, Missy! If I believed in an afterlife I'd join you."

Doug holds an empty glass up to Rafa, who shakes her head. He stows his bottle and the extra glasses, takes the wheel in one hand, and switches on the solar motor with the other. She sits on a wooden bench behind him as the boat glides out of the harbor and between the lighted buoys of the channel.

"Take the wheel," Doug commands.

Rafa asks, "Don't you want to raise the main sail?"

"That would take both of us. I don't have it in me. Bring up the turbines."

She takes the wheel and flips a switch that opens the hatch at the base of the main mast. A stack of demi-lunar wind turbines rises and spreads evenly, like the vertebrae of an extinct sea creature. The turbines spin and spin faster and faster until the boat is forming a cloud of high-pitched white noise. The forward end rises. Spray wets the deck.

She asks, "What's our heading?"

"South-southeast. We're going beyond the lighthouse at two o'clock."

She scans the horizon and finds a blue-white beacon. "Is that Pender?"

"North Pender Island. We're headed for Swanson Bay."

"Swanson? Is it named for Grandma?"

"As of last week."

"Who lives there?"

"Foraging and restoration guilders, a few healers, and no doc, of course."

Doug shouts over the white noise of the turbines, "Stop haunting me, Missy! Yes, I missed chances and made bad choices. Yes, I could have been a better man. But you can see it's too late."

Rafa adjusts their course. After a few minutes, the current pulls them east. She adjusts their heading again. "I can't remember how to measure the current."

Doug makes no reply. She calls to him, but he has passed out, and does not stir when she tries to wake him. She switches on the automatic pilot. Making her way below, she collects skins from the aft bunks and tosses them up the ladder. Climbing it with care, she covers Doug with two of the skins. Returning to the wheel, Rafa can't shake off the image of death gliding over the sea behind them, sickle propped on its shoulder, ready to take him for disrespecting the spirits of the ancestors. She is already missing Doug's skepticism, staunch friendship, and coyote-like delight in overturning order. She wonders if he had a grandma who was like that when she was old.

Rafa adjusts the boat's heading again. She loves the freedom and responsibility that come with being at the helm. She reaches out to catch the edge of the salt spray and tastes it. She crows and proves her freedom by heading toward each point of the compass in turn, going this way and that and then finally steering true. Soon she passes the lighthouse and senses the mouth of the bay off the starboard bow. Watching the imagers closely, she steers to a good anchoring place, lowers the turbines, shuts off the safety lights, and sets the anchor where the keel will not run aground.

The moon has set—or the fog has thickened. She is not sure which. She waits several minutes for her senses to adjust. Low waves lap gently against the stern. The boat rolls gently with the waves. The anchor line snaps taught. Rafa switches on the safety lights, grabs a fourfold sheepskin, and crawls onto the forward deck. She reaches the dinghy and uncovers and unties it. After a long and laborious interval of trial and error, she hoists it over the port side and releases it. Its bottom slaps the water.

Rafa realizes that she forgot to hold onto the line. She grabs a gaff from beneath the port rail and reaches toward the dinghy as her mind tries to construct a back-up plan. It is too late. To her relief, the gaff strikes something solid and she is able to hook the dinghy and bring it alongside. Holding the gaff in one hand, she takes out her pinlight to get a look at the dinghy. The maneuver saps her strength. She puts the pinlight away and tosses the sheepskin into the dinghy. She returns the gaff to its position, grips the port rail, waits for a trough, and lowers her body.

She catches the dinghy with her toes, finds the aft seat with her left foot, and releases the rail. She twists so as to land in the boat, but falls sideways on the seat. She wonders if the pains in her elbow and ribs signal broken bones. She is too winded and disoriented to remember the location of the mussel farm, or of the marker buoy that she saw on the imager. Her sense of place relies on the echoes from the surface of the water and Doug's boat.

After a few minutes, the dinghy collides with the boat. Rafa lifts her body onto the seat and finds the oar handles. She sets the oars in their locks. Her limbs work easily. She has no broken bones; the pains are from bruises. She pulls the oars and flushes a raft of migrating sea birds. She is maneuvering the dinghy around Doug's boat toward the mussel frames when her left oar strikes a buoy. She ties up there. All she needs to do is to keep the dinghy in the cove.

Rafa exhales in relief and hopes that the worst is over. Spreading one half of the skin over the bottom of the dinghy, she lies on it, covers her body with the other half and stares into the void above. She feels strangely calm and secure. No harm will come to her here. Death is not ready for her. She can't explain why, but she feels sure of it. As she puts her mind to her passions and aspirations, she drifts off to sleep.

4

Colette's Legacy

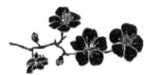

It seems to Sarah that nothing turns out as expected. The theater is packed with former students and followers of Randall and Colette who journeyed here from fertility and restoration schools around the polar circle and Pacific Rim. She knew that the two were well-loved; she didn't know she would have to scramble at the last minute to arrange two sets of repeated reenactments, and to host a spontaneous reunion with on-site encampment and an ad-hoc celebration that promises to go on for a month or more.

Nor did Sarah expect the state of joy of the community and its far-flung network to dispirit the group on stage. Behind her, John's mourning of Melissa is complicated by the enduring fire of his jealousy of Randall. Upstage, Aaron and Rafa are riding on adrenaline-fueled apprehension at the expected reenactment of an early and playful form of Randall and Colette's sacred sexual practice. Even Doug and Yukie seem out of sorts, perhaps because they have become more deeply engaged in mourning Melissa than they had intended. Parvati has already called Sarah's trio and Gina's wives to the stage to provide additional support for their key guests.

Sarah was also surprised at the unexpected degree of engagement expressed by some guests, which is pushing the boundary between order and disorder a bit too far toward chaos. The instance that she cannot get out of her mind is an old man from the far north asking Rafa—in all seriousness and with sincere expectation of prevailing—to have his baby. Another is that the bloodline advocates' desire to breed with Rafa and Aaron is set to become a serious problem. Leilani—with her Incan blood—has been talking about uniting the eagle and the condor—like the man from the north—or gathering Viking and Sephardic genes through Aaron's semen or through Rafa's eggs.

A spotlight comes up on Sarah. She begins, "Tonight, we will see the story of Randall and Colette, whose personal metamorphoses from profane to sacred sexual practices formed the core of our fertility teachings. If you have not yet taken sexual initiation, kindly return to the lodge for a day of games and skits. Not you, Rafa! This will serve as your formal initiation!"

A few young visitors gather around a performance guilder who is waiting beside the cycle block. As he leads the children to a trail that exits through the living alder wall, Sarah continues, "The action begins in Melbourne, Australia, where Colette has gone to stay with Reggie, who was then living with her extended family at Mount Macedon."

In the back row, a group of young men chant, "Aussie, Aussie, Aussie, oy, oy, oy," followed by a phrase taken from a Maori war chant. Sarah looks up to see a group she has heard about: a dozen indigenous Aussies and another dozen assorted young male Australians and New Zealanders with—rumor has it—a Tiwi Islander and a Papuan. They arrived on a sailboat that is now anchored in the harbor, and are on their way to a canoe racing tournament in Squamish. She has been meaning to seek them out and to find out what role they play in the fertility community, and whether it has anything to do with sport.

The lights go down. When the lights go up again, the action chronicles Colette's encounters with sacred and profane sexuality. First, she arrives in Melbourne and meets Reggie's childhood mates Liz and Ronnie, whose search for fleeting encounters in pubs disturbs Colette. Reggie offers to teach them all the rudiments of a redemptive sexuality.

Reggie freezes. A spotlight goes up on Colette, who turns to the audience and confesses, "I don't know how to explain how sex became my shame. I could tell her about my philandering relations, my obedient Catholic mother, the priest cousin who saw women as the root of all evil, the self-loathing teachings of nuns, or my self-subjugation to my husband Steve, who expected me to work harder than anyone else in exchange for my keep. But the problem is in here," she says, placing her palm over her pubic bone. "I let desire fester. I put off having children. And now I'm forty and single. Is this my chance to feel sexual joy, or will my shame deepen?"

Sarah can feel John's sorrow, and wonders if he is thinking of the lifelong friendship of Melissa and Colette, and of the likelihood that their early sexual formation was similar.

Colette continues in confused torment, "Is it right for me to shower my friend with troubles when she's giving me sanctuary? How can I be the friend I want to be? How—how can I be a woman, a lover, and a mother to vitality—mine and a man's? If I ask Reggie to hold these questions with me, will she understand and agree? She would have to know discernment as well as she knows joy. I shouldn't force familiarity. I should go slow!"

Colette turns to Reggie as the lights come up and Reggie unfreezes, and Colette says, "I don't know if I'll be equal to it."

"I'll be teaching sacred sexuality—very simply. If you want

to learn more, I can teach you to circulate and redirect energy, channel arousal—and stay cool around Andy."

Colette blushes, and says warily, "That sounds good."

"Look, Collo, I reckon you had a rough time with Steve. But that's over now. You're free to find your way—and to skip Andy. He's a married tomcat. He won't be able to leave you alone if he feels your longing."

Colette and the audience gasp as one, the audience apparently unaware of Andy's early sexual life. "I can resist him now that I know he's married."

"You can't. You have to know and own your energy, change your state so he senses no desire."

The lights go down. The audience converses. John asks Gina if they are talking about the founders, and if they are reluctant to stand and share unformed impressions of the founders' midlife struggles. Sarah takes the initiative. "Lights!" she says. When the lights have gone up she continues, "Would anyone like to comment on what they've just seen?"

An agro guilder stands and says, "This is a lot to take in. We didn't know that Reggie was the only one who practiced sacred sexuality at that time."

A fertility elder stands and says with relative serenity, "We haven't seen the founders surrounded by profane sexuality. We haven't seen them struggle with it. But we have seen the results of that struggle."

A hospitality guilder stands and says, "It's strange to see them acting like our students, or guests, or worse! I think of them as having always been wise."

"Good!" Sarah says. "Anyone else?"

Aaron says, laughing lightly, "I remember Mom going on

about Maimonides talking about women as if they were sexual toilets. She struggled with profane sexuality and became something of a renunciate."

John says, "I don't think you're being fair to our generation. Things were very different then, which brought out all kinds of change, including the change we're seeing now."

Rafa says, "Like changes in medicine."

Doug says, "Like changes we see everywhere but here."

Aaron looks at the audience, many of whom appear slightly stunned. It crosses his mind that they think too much alike, and are on the way to becoming a tribe unaware of its disconnection from the body of humanity.

Sarah says, "We can become a bit cloistered here—despite our connectivity. Thanks for the reminder, Doug. Lights!"

Several scenes later, as the friendship between Reggie and Colette deepens, a voice calls out from the audience, "I have a question for Parvati." A spotlight comes up on the stage audience as the crew continues a scene change upstage. A restoration elder stands and says, "We haven't seen Reggie express curiosity about Colette or anything else beyond her immediate concerns. I'd never seen her as self-satisfied, but there's something about it that rings true. Was it your intention to portray her that way?"

Parvati smiles. "Reggie was always preoccupied with the inner life—partly because she was working out how to translate and extract the teachings of her gurus. I wanted to show her transforming her inner life and allowing it to show through her being."

An agro elder stands and says, "The portrayals imply that Colette did the opposite—that she acted and let that show in her being. But she didn't. She also worked from the inside out."

A hospitality elder stands and says, "I agree—and that's

important. Colette surpassed her limitations to such a degree that we're free of them now."

Aaron asks, "What limitations were those?"

"In her spiritual work—which Reggie ignored because it had no practices for increasing control—Colette participated in peacemaking missions. She stood with and brought prayerful attention to indigenous peoples whose rights were being violated—usually by predation on the body of life."

"Do you mean to say that her peacemaking was a limitation?"

"Her limitation lay in perpetuating forces that polarize—dynamics like domination and submission. She took sides. She stood with the oppressed. All of us instinctively look beyond polarities to their source. We discern and reconcile oscillations and instabilities."

"Oscillations?"

"Contests between opposing forces—like control and helplessness. These can increase and lead to disruption and decay. We look at the full dynamic, discern the polarity—usually held by an unconscious habit—and reconcile it."

Aaron asks Parvati, "What was the reason you left out Colette's work?"

"I didn't realize that Reggie didn't move on as Colette did."

A fertility guilder stands and says, "I don't see that at all. Both women changed from the inside—Colette more than Reggie because Reggie was ahead of her from the start."

A hospitality guilder stands and says, "That remark proves the point. Reggie failed to see her limitations and so did we, so we perpetuated them. She and Graeme and all the founders focused on being over doing."

Gina says, "But we've joined being and doing with entrained

stances—like the ones Lena and Lisa and I teach in Vancouver. They prime us for fertile restoration, which is our great strength, and our greatest doing."

A performance guilder comes from center stage, kneels beside Sarah, and says, "I think what we're recognizing here is that we rely on the fertility and warrior guilds—and the restoration guild to some extent. That means that some guilds are more equal than others. And, we still have power dynamics."

Doug says, "He's right on the money. The fertility guild doesn't value doing as much as being, and the restoration guild has no group that develops new practices. You're holding fewer and fewer open questions. You're shorting rational inquiry and losing the contemplative sciences that evolve ideas and methods."

There is a deep silence. Sarah has the impression that the audience is stunned. She is glad when Doug continues, "I'd like to point out that Randall is the only one who seemed to take an interest in the body in its own right. He had a fine mind for clinical research, and went to Australia to develop surgical solutions for male infertility."

Aaron leans back and looks up at the sky as if seeking outside aid in discerning what is lacking. The audience remains silent.

Sarah laughs in delight, puts her hand on the actor's shoulder, and says, "Wonderful! This is the kind of breakthrough that Parvati sought through knowledge keeping, and that the performance guilders hoped to inspire in the enactments. And—and it sheds light on the struggles of Leilani and Siobhan, who may have sensed our incipient instability."

Parvati says, "This is too big a topic to discuss now, and what we see later may inform our discussion, so let's move on. Lights!" The lights go down.

Several scenes on, Colette encounters an extreme contrast between sacred and profane sex, the sacred taking the form of a sweet introductory teaching in tantric union that begins with gazing and loving speech, and the profane being a simultaneous orgy organized by Reggie's brother, Yanni, to thwart his sister, one that goes horribly wrong.

Sarah is surprised to feel John relax during this difficult scene, and soon hears him say to Gina, "The audience seems disgusted by profane sex."

Gina says, "We try to stay dispassionate, but we're averse to it."

"No naughtiness? No recreational release of pent-up tension?"

"We tend to our states at all times, and we're aroused by sacred union. Late modern sex makes no sense to us."

John squeezes her hand. "I'm glad you came here—and grateful to see what Randall accomplished here."

Sarah feels a lift of relief at John's posthumous reconciliation with Randall. Later, after a lunch break that Sarah spends with the stage audience in the private dining room, they return to the theater for the story of Randall and Colette's meeting and their rocky formation of the consort bond that led to the founding of the community and its network. After several scenes, Randall and Colette attend a Seder where Randall speaks almost as a rabbi-doctor, which causes their host to nickname him Maimonides. Afterward, they try a first union.

John asks Gina, "Will the actors, uh—join—onstage?"

"Probably. They belong to both the performance guild and the fertility guild. They're consorts and advanced practitioners—like Randall and Colette."

"I haven't felt arousal since your grandma died—a quarter

of a century ago."

"Did you and she … ?"

"We made love—literally. It helped. We did fine by modern standards."

Sarah feels a pang when she hears the regret in John's voice, and suspects that he is intensely aware that he and Melissa could have shared a consort practice had they returned here together after their first visit, as they had intended. He may even be thinking that Aaron's life might have been very different, or that Gina or Rafa might not have been born.

Sarah can feel the state of the theater audience unify and intensify spiritually and sexually as they relive the first union between two beloved founders and refresh the imprint of the consort bond that patterned—and lives on in—their community. On stage, the audience is quiet. Sarah, relieved and yet curious, steals glances at Rafa and Aaron and discovers that they are averting their eyes. Sarah smiles to herself; she need not have worried. They have avoided the problem of seeing more than they are ready to see.

Later, Sarah is pleased to hear the audience murmur in recognition of more evidence of Melissa's influence on Randall as well as Colette, and so on the formation of the whole community. The scene is a telephone call made by Randall to Melissa after Colette left him alone in Chicago as a result of Randall's workaholism, which pushed them into a crisis and divided them.

The actress playing Melissa, who is standing stage right talking into a phone, says, "You're at the edge of the abyss. Don't throw the past over the edge! Take its lessons. You helped bring new life into the world. You did plenty of things right—it's just that what's right is changing fast."

"Torah doesn't change."

"Interpretations do. With all the old and new knowledge of the world converging, they're going to change as never before."

"How do you know what to believe?"

"My body keeps me grounded, and honest. Does yours?"

"My gut is telling me to set up a fertility center where couples can share sensual and spiritual pleasures, and make love, and practice fertility the way the Chassids do on Shabbos—by returning to *Pardes*."

"Don't say that too loudly! You might be eaten alive by your own kind."

"You mean Jews?"

"I mean doctors."

Randall laughs darkly. "I almost wish I didn't know what I should do."

"You're ready to take life as your teacher. You know you won't learn the art of medicine from a computer. And you and I know better than John does that the art of medicine is a sacred one. The Rambam made it clear that we need both medicine and religion to care for the body. And so did Philip Tumulty."

"Who?"

"A clinician doctor. The one behind the teaching of clinical medicine as it was in our day—and today. There's been no progress since."

"Most modern medical traditions rely on dependence and deception. That came from medicine—and religion."

"We live in a time when we can hold ourselves to higher standards—spiritually and scientifically. We can face and delineate mistakes, reconcile our debts—and then move forward with life through time and place."

The audience murmurs, but no one speaks. John has the impression that they are noting that they can trace their core views back to Melissa.

Randall replies, "I want to follow Dr. Viktor Frankl. He came out of the Holocaust knowing that each of us had to discover our meaning and purpose and to act from them. I'm afraid to see what he saw—and afraid to look away."

"Is that why you kept Colette at arm's length?"

He doesn't reply.

"You're poised between the meaning of your past and the meaning you want to share with her. Choose that. Choose life." The lights go down.

Both Aaron and Rafa are attentive to the enactment of the dinner party during which the three founding couples—Andy and Lisa, Reggie and Graeme, and Colette and Randall—reveal to Reggie's friends that they have decided to express their fertility through their life work. Andy and Lisa will adopt degraded habitats and restore them to health, thereby modeling habitat adoption as a means of nurturing and perpetuating life on earth. Reggie and Graeme aim to develop exoteric and esoteric practices that will pattern the being, becoming, and doing of the community. Colette and Randall aim to teach fertility rather than to address infertility, and to evolve their teaching so as to encompass all kinds of offspring, which Colette is already calling thirds, and which include spirit and brain children and—in their case—a fertility community. Sarah hears Rafa say to Aaron, "Now I get what they do in concepto!" as the audience erupts in a cheer of celebration.

The audience murmur rises to a dull roar that quiets when the lights go up. Then the performance guilders reenact Randall's first, playful, ecstatic, shared embodiment of the tree of life as a template for sacred union—a template to this day taught in many variations by the fertility guilders. The theater audience is attentive and attuned and moved to joy and gratitude.

After the last scene, and after the applause dies away, Sarah asks that the lights dim and the audience reflect on the enactment for five minutes. Then, the lights come up on Sarah again, who says with joy, "We all know that Randall called on his former patient Mac, that Mac provided this land, and that the founders created this community—and we know how it has grown and evolved so far!"

A hospitality guilder stands and says, "I don't like to even think this, but I don't think we'd be here if Yanni hadn't done what he did. Colette and Reggie and all the others were too preoccupied and too complacent."

An agro guilder stands and says, "Reggie didn't accept what was going wrong until things spun out."

A fertility guilder says, "Those of us who are caught up in being forget about doing—and vice versa."

An agro guilder says, "We all know that if we practice union too often and too long we think of energy and forget matter."

Sarah adds, "Remember: it's natural to feel some distress after seeing a conflict. Our bodies imbibe it and mirror it and it works in us for some time."

Parvati says, "I think that what they're saying is that they feel a need for something that we saw and that we generally dismiss. Juxtaposition, disagreement, and conflict accomplishes things that we may not be accomplishing now."

Doug says, "What do the warriors have to say?"

Oke Ten rises. "I will speak for our guild. Conflict is not the issue; avoidance is the issue. Most of us want to be comfortable, and we can be. As warriors, we are often uncomfortable, and come to value the discomfort that signals uncertainty and risk."

Aaron asks, "Is there a particular guild that hangs back?"

"Fertile restoration is going well, and yet still too slowly." Oke Ten sits.

Aaron is not sure of Oke Ten's intent. "Are you saying that the community is losing its potency?"

Oke Ten does not reply.

Belatanu says pointedly, "We value dialogue until it becomes difficult."

Doug says, "The only real obstacle to progress for anyone—or any group—is thinking you've got it all figured it out. That's the primary cautionary tale of modern times."

Kim says, "If we're only interested in ourselves—if we're incurious or biased or set in our ways, we'll leave nothing but our ashes."

Parvati says, "We're moving into knowledge keeping—which the performance guild is holding with fabro design. We're developing our doing between guilds."

Rafa says, "You don't have any knowledge creators—no experimentalists or explorers."

Sarah says, "Let's wrap this up for now and meet in the sanctuary to continue this dialogue after dinner—after we've had time to think and before we've become complacent!"

5

Disruptors

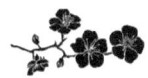

The next afternoon, a horse-drawn cart bounces down a leaf-strewn track from the agro center to the orchards. Rafa finds the seemingly romantic ride jolting and tiring. It doesn't help that she is packed onto the cart's bare wood seats with two dozen other initiates and stacks of supplies. She jumps down and walks behind the cart. Belatanu, Léon, and Dirk jump out after her.

Belatanu asks Rafa, "So, are you going to be a woman of the field or of the sea?"

"I can't tell if that's a serious question."

"Think of it this way," Léon says, "We choose up teams by habitat."

"Teams?"

Belatanu says, "Every being belongs to at least one habitat. We belong to several, so we choose one to live or work in and call it our own. Most fertility guilders choose forest. Most agro guilders choose field."

Rafa says, "Today I'm a woman of the field. So tell me what that means."

"Oh, no!" Léon says. He pulls Dirk by the arm and the two of them rush past the wagon and out of earshot of Belatanu, who expatiates on the wonders of human-created habitats. As they emerge from the forested hill and look out over the fecund fields that extend to Fulford Harbor, Belatanu points out curving rows of berry bushes enclosed by an earthen dam; diagonal rows of pear, apricot, and cherry trees; and rows of apple trees. Every bit of earth is used to grow crops on several levels, which gives it the appearance of one big garden.

Rafa enjoys the wide open skies. She would like to enjoy the forest the way Doug does—as a part-time resident. But Belatanu's passion for the fields is contagious. These musings are cut short when the cart stops, the clean-up teams descend, and an agro elder climbs up on the cart to give them instructions.

Rafa listens and looks at the fruit trees. They are short and bare, and the withering herbs and bare shrubs below them reveal compost and soil. Ducks, sheep, and goats have dotted the ground with scat. When the elder finishes explaining how to prune and spread mulch, the four friends go to the end of a nearby row of trees and help themselves to the materials that the agro elders put there. Each takes a green flax apron with ample front pockets along with pruning shears, a pitch fork, a shovel, or a wheel barrow. Belatanu breaks them into pairs to spread mulch or to prune trees and cut back shrubs.

When Rafa and Léon have pruned their first row, and Belatanu and Dirk—who have been hauling the mulch—catch them up, they switch tasks and go around the compost fence to return along the next available row.

"How does this work?" Rafa asks, pointing to the empty composting fence, which is formed by two rows of thatched fencing. Dirk says, "In the spring, we fill it with mixed grasses, clover, and other compostables, and in the summer it sprouts long, thick grasses that the livestock eat; then, in the fall, we spread it on the ground.

"So how did you like the enactment?" Dirk asks.

"I'd call it strange and wonderful."

"No terrors, or ghosts?" Léon asks eagerly.

"I won't get to those for a long time. Syncing is in my future."

The others tease Rafa about how far in the past she is living, after which Léon asks boldly, "So, Rafa, are you looking for a consort?"

Rafa stops and looks at Léon. His face is filled with desire. Rafa has never seen a man look at her like this. Unexpectedly, her body responds. She looks away in confusion and picks a few apples. "Is that … an invitation?"

"Yes."

"I thought you liked me."

"I do."

"Not a good idea."

"I agree," Léon says lightly. Desire disappears from his face.

She says ironically, "I'm disappointed by your lack of disappointment."

"I was interested, too," Dirk says casually, "but Sarah said I only felt that way because you're new and don't want anything from me."

Belatanu says, "Your energy is still all over the place. You're confusing everyone. You're mine!"

Rafa deadpans, "I can't tell you how flattered I feel."

Léon says edgily, "Belatanu's center is so intense that he can shine the sun of bliss on anyone and take all their troubles away."

Dirk laughs.

"Why is that funny?" Rafa asks.

Dirk says, "Léon's implying that Belatanu is playing

power games, which opens the door to controlling, which is Neanderthal."

"Léon!" Belatanu says, "That's enough."

Rafa feels a wave of desire. She looks at Léon and feels the pull of his eyes, and then looks away and shifts uncomfortably.

Belatanu says irritably, "Don't play with Rafa like that! You have no manners."

Léon wheedles, "You know how confused I am right now."

"I know you're taking advantage of it. If you want to stay out of your hammock you'd better not link sex with force!"

"What's going on?" Rafa asks in alarm.

"Manipulative or coercive union is a crime against community," Belatanu says solemnly. "We don't bypass rites—for good reasons."

Rafa feels the tension between Belatanu and Léon. Léon relents and relaxes into Belatanu's strength. His energy descends and grounds his body in the earth. Belatanu releases him. They go back to picking.

Rafa says, "It felt like you were controlling him."

"I was using sanctioned, purposeful controlling that Léon asked for and that I agreed to provide to him so he could get out of his hammock."

Léon sighs heavily. "I just … can't … control myself."

"You'll be fine right now if you leave Rafa to me."

Léon nods morosely.

Belatanu looks Rafa in the eye. He is seeking her consent. She smiles shyly and nods. He says, "Rafa and I committed to a one year consortship."

"About time," Léon says excitedly, as if filled with the news and eager to tell everyone.

"Now you're syncing," Dirk says to Rafa with a grin. He adds in a whisper, "And now we can tell you what we've been afraid to. You and *Tío* have to watch out for Leilani and Siobhan."

Rafa knocks on her uncle's door. *Tío* opens it; on seeing her, he smiles warmly and gestures toward the desk chair. It's her first time in this room, which like hers, is in the wing reserved for family guests. They have a bed, desk and desk chair, shelves, and a closet. There is enough floor space for yoga or meditation. There are wall hooks and a cork board. Tío has hung nothing and the shelves are empty but for a few samples of plants and sand-smoothed shells.

Rafa says the words she has rehearsed. "We're kin already, and becoming kind."

Tío's eyebrows shoot up. "This sounds serious."

Rafa gathers her thoughts, studies her uncle's face, and says, "I've heard a disturbing rumor. I don't know what to do. I want your advice."

Aaron's face registers surprise and then concern. "Go on."

"It has to do with Leilani and Siobhan."

Aaron shakes his head. "Are they flirting with you now?"

"Word is they're planning to drug you—and steal your seed."

Aaron's eyebrows shoot up. "Are you sure?"

"I'm sure there's a rumor. The guys told me that they also intend to control and sedate me and steal my eggs, and that we should use a buddy system and lock the door at night."

"That's cloak and dagger. Were they teasing you? Hoaxing you?"

"I don't think so."

Aaron frowns pensively. "We should try and talk with Sarah."

He rises and leads Rafa out of his room, down the stairs, and down the hall to Sarah's. He listens attentively and then knocks softy. After a pause, Parvati opens the door and waves them in. Sarah is curled up on the bed in her white robes with her cane hooked over the head of the bed. Yuko and Parvati are tending to her. Rafa realizes that Sarah is showing how close she is to the end of her life every day—in private.

Aaron says, "Rafa heard a rumor that may require a response."

When they are seated, Yuko-Hyun asks them to wait while she brings Sarah's support team. Sarah sighs and closes her eyes. Soon the door opens and Yukie enters with Selah, Dora, and Ella, who take up places between the bed and the wall opposite the line of chairs.

Aaron looks at Rafa, who repeats the conversations she had with her friends in the apple orchard. When she finishes Sarah says irritably, "Je-Sus! I am fed up with the two of them! The plot you describe violates our core principles. We have no choice but to hold a trial. I should have seen that Leilani needed to be elsewhere. I want you to sleep on the floor of your uncle's room. Can you do that? You can spend your waking hours with Aaron, or Björn, or Doug, or Belatanu—until the trial."

"Got it."

"Stay with me now and let me tell you stories about your grandma. When I'm done, you can go and join your uncle."

Later on, when Aaron has climbed into bed and Rafa is lying on a pile of skins at its foot, she says, "I did the fabro trader initiation project by designing a clinic building that will lead into my vocation project, and I want to make and sell the buildings as my vocation. I want to include Bel's herb garden, and I want to include teams, which would tie it into your legacy project."

Aaron whistles softly. He turns out the overhead lights and turns on a strip of green pinlights as night lights. "That's ambitious."

"It's like Oke Ten said, things come together and open a way ahead."

Aaron laughs softly, deep in his throat. "Let's hear the specifics."

Rafa says, "I want to build the prototype clinic in the fabro center and move it up to the road, and sell it to a hot springs spa up-island that Yukie told me about. Then I want you to recruit a team from the Amanas to come and staff it. After it gets going, I want to make clinic structures for export that support the kind of medicine Grandma did. I could start a new guild."

"Did you talk with Björn and Doug about this?" Aaron asks doubtfully.

"Yes."

"Sure. We should talk through the feasibility and workplan. But not now."

"I want to ask you something else," Rafa says pensively. "Grandma and Grandpa were doctors, and Dad was a psychologist, and you worked for a clinic. Do you think I was born to do something in medicine?"

"We've done enough for medicine. Do it only if you can't not do it."

"I can do without it. What about you? What's your project?"

"Well, so far all I know is that I must face the unknown—in this case, unknown problems that limit the future of this community. That means looking for a lack and its roots. I think that the ultimate problem has something to do with syncing with life in place and time, but I'm not sure."

"Why syncing?"

"They're small, and they're focused. They progress far and fast in certain areas—like fertile restoration—but neglect others."

"Like what?

"Medicine and religion, for starters. They can only support so many guilds, so they have no doctors or clergy. Your project would help with that."

"They'd have the right kind of clinic nearby. And those who want to could join congregations on the island."

"That might do—if our community accepts that they don't know as much as they think they do about contemplation or science, or for any other way of holding open-ended questions and looking for new solutions. No one here could have a conversation with the likes of Maimonides, or Darwin, or Einstein."

"They wouldn't want to. Yukie teaches the kids that the Middle East is nothing but oil and nuclear barrens now because Jews were imprinted by Nazis, which made Einstein create nuclear weapons."

Aaron groans. "Turning away from the wisdom of science will undo Mom's core teachings and turn back the clock. This community is so intent on the foreground of creation that the universe is a blur to them. They don't even network with field scientists like mycologists and plant pathologists. They don't think about water tables or soil deficiencies or partial pressures of oxygen. The oxygen levels have fallen to what they used to be at 7200 feet and could fall further. They need to be tracking that and preparing to adapt—now and from now on."

Rafa is enjoying the conversation. She can talk more easily with *Tío* now than with anyone else. "If bloodlines don't matter, why is it so easy for me to talk to you—now that I know you, I mean?"

"Our parents probably imprinted our shared characteristics on us in the womb, and in infancy, which brings us back to Grandma."

"They expect so much of us—you especially. I don't want to be a tick, but I don't want to do more than we should. Belatanu is worried that we're burning out."

"We shouldn't do too much for them or we'll coopt their processes and set them up for domination, and that would—" Aaron's voice goes up at the end, cuing Rafa to say with him, "turn back the clock." They laugh quietly. Aaron asks, "What's a tick?"

"Someone who sucks resources without giving back—and spreads seeds of illness."

Soon, Aaron begins to snore. Rafa smiles, turns on her side, and goes to sleep.

Belatanu drops his wheelbarrow on the matted grass of the winter pasture, wipes his brow, and exclaims incredulously, "You told Sarah about Leilani!"

Rafa's heart sinks. "What's wrong with that?"

"We never tell her things like that. We tell Parvati, and she and Yukie figure out how to tell Sarah."

Rafa snorts and grins. "How is *Tío* supposed to solve that problem?"

"Why would he?"

"That's what Sarah wants from him, isn't it?"

"We handle things like that personally. This is a family. We all make it work."

"You do not. The bloodline problem went on too long. Remember what Oke Ten said about avoidance?"

"We had it under control."

"Did you?"

Belatanu crosses his arms, sighs heavily, and says reluctantly, "I don't know. What I know is that we wanted to spare Leilani's children, and that we can't do that now."

"How would it be for them if she raped me or *Tío*?"

Belatanu's shoulders sink. "Leilani thinks that flesh generates the body, and that successful long-term adaptation depends on genes. We can't afford to ignore that point of view."

"Kim said that Leilani is a disruptor, not a dissenter."

"She always says that, but no one else can see it. Siobhan didn't. It's almost as if she's a—she's a—"

"She's a what?"

"Well, if it's going to trial, it'll come out, so I may as well say." Belatanu sighs. "Siobhan may be an empty."

"An empty?"

"A person who invites domination."

"I can't imagine Leilani needing an invitation."

"Siobhan's pull is strong. She more than encourages Leilani."

"If you saw it coming, why did it get so far?"

"Here, each of us is always balancing being and interbeing. We try to create a strong core—and a strong community. That pulls us in opposite directions—in and out. We need room to struggle and make mistakes. That means keeping things informal and unstructured. Leilani took advantage of the situation, Siobhan aggravated it, and our mistakes perpetuated it. Yes, there's a problem, but things don't always go just right. I don't think we did anything wrong."

"Maybe it had to come to this. I can see that you did something wrong, and I think you can see it if you try."

"With all due respect, neither you nor Aaron knows our ways."

"With all due respect, she didn't want your seed, she wanted mine, and I don't see what Sarah could have done about that, especially if you didn't even tell her. Plus, Sarah and her friends won't be around much longer and all that will remain is *Tío's* legacy. You should figure out what you want and tell him."

He sighs. "Okay, point taken."

"And tell me what I can do to make it easier."

"You can ask Yuko-Hyun to look out for Leilani's family. There's going to be a scandal, and then a trial, and then our detractors will use all that against us. And she can't let the wrong person or group get hold of Leilani. Leilani knows how to hurt us—and she's not a very attentive mother."

Rafa feels as if her ribs have frozen in place. "She might act against her own children? Why don't you say so at the trial—or speak for her and her family?"

"You won't mind if I speak against you?"

"No—if it helps you figure things out and work it through."

Belatanu nods thoughtfully. "It all depends on Leilani's consort—what he wants as a consort and what he decides as an initiator and a warrior."

"I thought you didn't know who the initiators were!"

"I should learn that I can't talk freely around you!"

"Or you should talk to me so that I can point out the problems that get past you."

After a long, frowning pause, Belatanu says quietly, "Fair enough. The point I was making about her consort is that he's a complex-any—unpredictable, and so creative that no one understands his practices. He's so good with the unknown and unseen that Sarah gave him the name Wind Carver. He's developed the ability to put himself in the shoes of any malefactor or fool, and to circumvent any obstacle that anyone might put in our way. If he decided to use that against us ... "

"Do you mean he'd take her side against everyone else?"

"I mean that he isn't a member of the community—he is the community. That's one reason Sarah doesn't send him on missions. If we lost him, we'd be left without an essential piece of ourselves. That's true of every loss, of course, but losing him would mean losing our core. It would set us back."

"This sounds like something *Tío* should know."

"You're right. We should be talking to him, telling him the things we take for granted—or avoid—until something happens and we have to take a good look at ourselves."

Aaron scans the crowd in the Forest Sanctuary. The room is so packed that he is sweating even though it is cold out, and even though the warriors who are forming the inner and outer perimeters have retracted all the glass walls so as to seat newcomers in the gardens outside. As it fills all the way to the forest, he guesses that the majority of the enactment guests have come to the trial. He also sees outside guests: Jerome Beaulieu III, the town mayor, the town communicator. Even families with small children have come and are filling up a triangular cry room made of glass panels. Most community members are wearing formal clothes, as are the schoolers, pre-initiates, and initiates seated around Aaron and Parvati. He doesn't see Rafa, and concludes that she is outside with Yuko-Hyun.

Aaron feels undercurrents of anger, sorrow, excitement,

aggression, tension, aversion, and fear. Parvati is actively transforming these hell states into fertile ones; he is sharing a strong care state with her. Sarah is already seated on the central platform opposite Leilani and Siobhan. Behind Leilani stands Wind Carver, who is tall and muscular and has symmetrical, broad features set in a mask of self-contained pride. Aaron guesses that the girl and two boys standing beside him are his children. The family is gorgeous; beside them, Siobhan and her fine-looking consort and fidgety children look ordinary.

A gong sounds outside. Respectful attentiveness blankets the sanctuary and stills the energy. Sarah says, abruptly and dispassionately, "Leilani, you are accused of controlling and domination. Who will speak for you?"

Leilani says self-righteously, "No one. I have no regrets."

Wind Carver places his hand lightly on her shoulder. She relaxes and continues, "My actions speak for me. For years I tried to make you see that we lack strong bloodlines. I took responsibility for it by breeding my own. We tried to persuade the solitary son and granddaughter of the new founders to share seed, but they have other plans. So I conspired to continue their bloodlines in spite of all of you, and I ask you to listen to us, follow us, and reward us."

Parvati whispers in distress, "They're trying to control Sarah!"

"How do you know?"

"I feel their laser focus! They're stronger than I knew."

"Can you help Sarah?"

"Wait—there's a change. Do you feel that?"

"It feels ... calmer—peaceful."

"Look at the warriors. They've closed their eyes and adopted a practice pose. They're diverting energy from control to reconciliation!"

"Who will protect her?"

"They're already doing it by converting the energy of the accused—and by using whatever energy they draw from their guild."

"Why is Sarah just sitting there? Are they controlling her?"

"I don't know."

After a pregnant pause, Sarah says, "Witnesses say that you conspired to steal a man's and a woman's seed by force, and so to cut the threads of goodwill that form the fabric of our peace, and to intercept our sacred, shared purpose for your narrow-minded, self-willed, short-sighted, and spurious ends. This constitutes controlling, a crime against community. Just now, you abused your practice by trying, in this sacred place, to impose your will on mine. All of the advanced practitioners present in the sanctuary can bear witness to your attempt at domination, which is an intangible crime against community."

"It is a sacred practice by which we intend to save the community from you," Leilani counters.

"The wellbeing of each is the wellbeing of all. You cannot save your own body or any body, individual or shared, by giving form to fears and forcing others to submit to them. You can only save your body, and other bodies, by owning and transforming fears. You had every chance to learn this and all our ways. Instead, you became enchanted with fixed ideas and closed your inner and outer eyes to all we hold dear."

"So you say."

"You will have one more chance to learn," Sarah declares. "That chance is banishment. You will have three hours to pack a bag for yourself and leave alone. Four warriors will escort you. From the time you leave our perimeter and for the next five years, any warrior who sees you within five miles of this lodge, or any advanced practitioner who detects you breaking into the group mind, or any graduate, friend, or associate of this community who sees you nearing this place, or hears of you planning to do so, will alert the warriors, who will remove you to a place from which you will find it very difficult to return."

Leilani looks contemptuous, and then confused, and finally enraged. Her exquisite features form fierce lines of hate.

Sarah continues, "When five years are up, if you accept your time debt and wish to return to reconcile it, you may send a request and the community will consider it. If they approve, you can return for a trial period."

"You old witch!" shrieks Leilani. She stands and rants, "You can't make the rules forever! You can't immortalize your views! You've tried to rewrite our history and turn us over to outsiders, but when you die, which will be soon, we'll recognize the primacy of flesh and teach the continuity of bloodlines!"

"Sit down!" Sarah commands.

Wind Carver places his hand lightly on Leilani's shoulder. She sits resentfully.

Sarah scans the group. The restoration guilders look crestfallen; the fertility guilders project compassion; and the warriors bow their heads as if acknowledging loss of respect due to the involvement of Leilani's consort.

Sarah continues, "I am grateful that Pea didn't live to see you undo her legacy! Contemplate her strength, your malice against life, and the consequences of your malice to your consort and all your relations." Sarah lifts her hand. The gong sounds. She turns to Leilani's sister and says gently but firmly, "Siobhan! I accuse you of being an empty."

Sarah pauses. The loving nurturance of the fertility guild fractures. Discord rises like a miasma. Confounded whispers collide like distracted thoughts in a diseased body. Aaron hears phrases like 'I thought so!' and 'I had no idea!' and 'She could say that about any of us!' and 'What about Aaron and Rafa?' and 'Who will be next?'

The murmuring dies down. When the room is silent and the crowd rapt, Sarah continues, "You lost interest in the work of becoming, which is the central responsibility of adult membership. You relied more and more on interbecoming and submitted more and more to a willful sister. Your inner vacuum increased and invited controlling. This undermined our consensus and depleted our shared purpose."

Aaron feels discord turning to concord.

Sarah asks, "Who will speak for you?"

Siobhan looks serene and trusting, and then fearful, and then bereft. Her delicate beauty becomes a blank. "I used to speak for myself. I should do that. I saw that the community was betraying its purpose. I remember that. I thought that bloodlines might be our salvation—especially with our genetic adaptation to high altitude. But the old reality is gone and the new ... is too."

"Was your sister controlling your being?"

"We were afraid that our lineage would end. We wanted to enhance the vigor of our bloodline to ensure continuation."

"What do you think of Leilani's plan to steal seed?"

"If the web of life dies, all bloodlines will end," Siobhan answers. "Here ... now ... I can't see how we put our ideas before that, or before being ... or becoming."

"Was the group controlling you?"

"My trust in a higher power prevents that," Siobhan says abruptly, and with surety.

Leilani stands and snarls, "There is no higher power!"

Siobhan appears stricken.

Sarah declares to Leilani, "Sit down and remain silent!"

Wind Carver again puts his hand on Leilani's shoulder. After a brief inner struggle, she complies.

Sarah frowns. After a long pause, she asks carefully, "Did you deify your beliefs, or your sister's beliefs?"

"I don't know … what do you mean?"

Parvati whispers to Aaron, "Sarah suspects that Wind Carver and Siobhan's consort Raven Rapper may have instigated the crime—and involved their children! Idolatry—creating an illusion to deny fears of the unformed—is usually a group error. It's difficult for an individual—or pair—to sustain it."

Aaron looks at the warriors standing on the inner perimeter. They look upset. The trial is taking a heavy toll on their guild.

"You know them," he whispers to Parvati. "What do you think?"

"I think the children will be fine if they stay with us."

"Siobhan," Sarah repeats, "did you put your beliefs about the primacy of the flesh above all else? Did you adore those beliefs, or fear to question them?"

"We may have … made metal … of sacred living waters."

Sarah sighs in apparent relief. "Are you saying that you held fixed ideas that limited your being or becoming?"

"We felt safe," Siobhan says with piteous perplexity. "But now I don't know why."

Sarah sinks in her seat and, after a pause, states sadly but resolutely, "Siobhan, you chose to become an empty. Your inner vacuum attracted controlling. When your sister planned to steal seed, you acted passively. You did not dissuade her or inform us. You abandoned your responsibilities and forfeited your membership in the community. You are hereby suspended."

Sarah lifts her hand. The gong sounds. She stares fixedly at Wind Carver. He does not speak. She says sadly, "Wind Carver. Your consort conspired to steal the seed of honored guests. You must have known of her enchantment with bloodlines and of her plans to use force. You did not discourage her, or alert others. How do you plead?"

After a heavy pause, he asks, "Are you accusing me of a thought crime?"

Sarah frowns and examines him under her brows. "If we discover in our bodies or in any aspect of our interbeing any intent to break a vow or to commit a crime against the community, we are bound to actively prevent the crime. To do otherwise is to aid and abet it. Did you abet either crime?"

"In our union, I adored Leilani, and she persuaded me to value bloodlines."

"Did you know of her plan to steal seed?"

"No."

"How can this be?"

"After her first conception we created a practice that protected the privacy of sacred seed gathering."

"It allowed her to breed, and blinded you to her acts of breeding?"

Wind Carver frowns. "In hindsight, yes."

"Will you uphold your responsibilities from now on?"

The room is so still that it seems to Aaron that no human is breathing, nor any animal within a hundred yards. Wind Carver looks to the warriors. None will meet his eyes. Finally, he says, "Yes."

Relief passes over Sarah's face. She asks, "Raven Rapper, how do you plead?"

"Leilani talks. She talks and talks and talks and does nothing. I never believed that she would do any of the things she was talking about."

Sarah says sharply, "She has borne children by several fathers. She has pursued seed with increasing urgency. She has become obsessed. She spoke of using force. Your decision to ignore all danger appears to be unreasoning complacency or careless disregard. Both are at odds with the mission of the warrior guild. Did anyone encourage you in this?"

"I was spending as little time as possible with my consort and her sister."

"You neglected your relations. What is your view of bloodlines?"

"Everyone has one and has to adapt to it. It's foolish to breed humans. That assumes that we're superior to the web of life, or can foresee the ramifications of breeding a complex species."

"How did you respond to Siobhan's choice to cultivate bloodlines?"

"I didn't like it. Siobhan did what Leilani wanted over my objections."

"How do you view her children?"

"They are hers, and they are not to blame for it, so they are mine."

"How will you care for them in her absence?"

"The way I do now."

"I see. Who will plead for the children?"

"I will," Parvati says. She stands, looks at the children, and chooses her words carefully. "The consort work of Leilani and Wind Carver has been so hot that the children felt compelled to take sides. All took shelter with their father. During the day, they study in school and do well; in the evening they teach habitat restoration to fertility students and do well."

"They teach?"

"Any of our children can teach visiting adults."

"What will they need to recover from their mother's banishment?"

"The same thing they need now; a personal, reliable maternal bond."

"And Siobhan's children?"

"The consort work of Siobhan and Raven Rapper has been so cold that the children have bridged the union to care for both parents. They spend their days in school and do well, and most evenings in the forest hunting with their father or gathering herbs with their mother."

"What will they need to recover from their mother's suspension?"

"They would benefit from each parent forming a strong consort practice that makes space for the children to grow in love as thirds."

"You recommend the dissolution of failed consortships and the formation of fertile new unions?"

"Yes, for the sake of the children and community as well as those who failed in their core responsibilities as adult members."

"Permission to speak!" calls a stern voice.

Sarah responds formally. "The third Jerome Beaulieu has the floor."

He stands. Aaron recognizes him as Jerome Junior's son, who Doug calls Jerbeau. He is wearing the ceremonial garments of his Vancouver sect, which traces its lineage to a guru in the Indus. The garments include a blue turban, a white silk sheath and pantaloons, and a splendid fuchsia and purple vest embroidered with pearls and quartz. Over all of this, he wears a floor-length, long-sleeved robe of the same material. Aaron can see, tucked into the top of his blue kidskin moccasins, the haft of a bone knife encrusted in mother of pearl. Jerbeau's expression is fierce and his posture is imposing. "I will take the banished Leilani as my consort."

Leilani turns toward him, mouth agape.

Parvati whispers, "He knows her well. She loves show. She will be captivated by his fine looks."

Aaron looks at Wind Carver, whose silky black hair falls thickly over his shoulders to his waist and sets off his broad, fit build and wide, confident stance. His perfectly proportioned features and fine posture seem to lift him above other men. Jerbeau appears to Aaron to be Wind Carver's equal.

Sarah asks skeptically, "Have you no concern about her love of power?"

"I have strong practices," Jerbeau replies confidently, adding respectfully, "but would ask someone from this community to observe her progress."

"Have you no concerns that she may hatch a scheme to harm your group?"

Jerbeau shakes his head and says, "Here, each of you works from the core. Each of you takes responsibility for developing discipline and creativity in pursuit of fertility. All share these processes and guide group action. In other words, you work from the inside out.

"We work from the outside in. Our leaders impose uniform, tangible, prescribed practices that accord with scripture and tradition. We offer a structure that can rule those who—like Leilani—lack the discipline and creativity to rule themselves. Those who can rule themselves are free to do so provided they surrender to our codes and leaders, who in turn surrender to our heritage. We expect this to suit Leilani and so we expect to rule her easily."

"Have you no concern that she may violate your codes?"

"If she does, she will take the consequences. If she were to steal a man's seed, I would slit her throat."

Sarah says sternly, "That is unacceptable to me. She can go with you only if you agree to respect the sanctity of life. Should she violate your codes, you can return her to us—without harm. Is that acceptable to you?"

Jerbeau stares at Leilani. After a few moments, she looks away. He says, "We will ensure her safety and accept a decision as to her punishment if it is made by one representative of this community and one appointed by our council."

"That is acceptable to me," Sarah says. "Leilani, what say you?"

"Would you allow me to continue my practices?" she asks Jerbeau.

"I would encourage you to follow the standard practices of this community. I wish to learn your ways of union and to adapt them for my sect."

"What rights will I have as your consort?"

"You will be my wife and subject to my will, unless you choose to leave and return to this community."

"Subject to your will?" she retorts disdainfully.

"Your body and being would be yours. I would take them as they are. Your doing would belong to me and to my sect. If you act with love, honor, and respect you will have no problem."

Leilani ponders. She does not consult her sister or children or consort. Finally she asks, "Will you … give me your seed?"

"I chose sterility. I cannot give it to you and you cannot steal it."

"You are disrespecting your ancestors!" she says hotly.

He smiles slightly. "I am fulfilling their purpose. You are fulfilling nothing. Our greatest human weaknesses are not of the flesh."

Leilani stares at Jerbeau long and hard. He stares back with intense confidence. Parvati whispers, "She's trying to control him and he won't let her." A minute later, Leilani says, "I respect you and will go with you."

"Before I give permission, I have another question for Jerbeau," Sarah says. "Domination foments secrets and subterfuge. Might your sect encourage her new habit of scheming?"

"The council, which has sanctioned this union, will watch us carefully."

After a long pause, Sarah asks hesitantly and hopefully, "Will anyone take Siobhan?"

"I will," Léon says. He stands to full height and expands his chest. "I will take her for a trial year of remote habitat restoration."

The crowd stirs. Aaron hears murmurs of surprise and disbelief. He can see now that Jerome's offer was anticipated—and that Léon's was not.

"Why will you?" asks Sarah, dubiously.

He replies with a touch of bravado. "I won't be able to empty her and she won't be able to use my interbeing. We will both have a chance to recover."

Parvati whispers, "That's very brave. I'm sure that anyone who felt impelled to partner her is glad he stepped up!"

"What about your declaration?" Sarah asks.

"I declared as a simple-same, but I've been feeling confused, and complex."

"Haven't we all?" Sarah replies skeptically.

"I've been talking with the counselor about it. I feel different when she grounds me."

Sarah says to the room, "Can anyone confirm this?"

The fertility guilder sitting beside him says, "Yes. It seems that his interbeing was very unstable, and that his poor grounding compromised his declaration. He seems to have been an oral sex addict and not a simple-same. When he is grounded, he is aroused by me and—it seems—by her. I would advise him to redeclare as a complex-diff."

"Give that to me as a Kinsey score."

"Somewhere between four and six."

Aaron hears scattered conversation. Sarah raises one eyebrow, sighs heavily, and asks, "What say you, Siobhan?"

"He is young... but old enough to have fathered my children."

Sarah shakes her head. "Not by mutual consent. Think before you speak."

Siobhan turns to Raven Rapper, who looks away. For a moment, she looks as if she might cry, and then she blurts, "I want to go with Leilani."

"You can't," Sarah says.

Siobhan looks at Léon, who smiles invitingly and appears to delight in her. "I want to go with him—if my children can come with me."

"Raven Rapper will take full responsibility for the children until your restoration is well under way." Sarah says, and then asks, "What will you do to restore your core processes of being, becoming and doing?"

"I don't know!"

"Who will speak for Siobhan?"

"I will," Parvati says. She stands and continues, "Siobhan was a very strong student. In her last years of school, when Leilani shifted to the fertility center, Siobhan did strong projects on habitat restoration. She could continue them as she rewrites her personal narrative."

Sarah says, "Take a minute and think back on those projects. Could you do one now?"

Siobhan frowns. After a pause, she says, "Our surface water is still unclean in some places. I could test plants to see if any of them will purify it and catalyze succession. Or I could do that someplace else where the water is dirtier."

A fertility guilder stands. He has a shaven head with a high, shiny crown. "Her being and energy are strong. We could teach them a safe consort practice and devise a practice to strengthen her becoming and doing and his interbeing."

A restoration guilder stands. "That project is of interest to us. We could guide their restoration."

"Good," Sarah says decisively. She asks for consorts for the others. Kim offers to take Wind Carver and Cookie volunteers to take Raven Rapper. Both offers are accepted. Sarah smiles with astonished relief, and says, "Léon, Kim, and Cookie, be aware that you are taking responsibility for any subtle or tangible use of controlling or domination or submitting by your consorts, and for any use of force or plans to use force. Do you accept this responsibility knowingly and gladly?"

"Yes," they reply.

"Good!" Sarah says. "Now! Now ... the community also played a role in these crimes. Our complicity lay in aiding and abetting the transgressors by delaying intervention until it was too late to sustain consort and family bonds. Who will speak for us?"

"I will," says Björn, standing above the rows of fabro workers.

"How do you plead?"

"I think it was unavoidable. If we were too quick to intervene, we'd limit learning, conscience, and creativity. We learn from our errors whether or not we're doing the right thing. From now on, we can look out for disruptors."

"So you think we drew the line in the right place—at the use of force. Anyone else?"

Belatanu stands. "I could have spoken up earlier, but I had got into the habit of stopping the flow of unpleasant information. I should speak up so that Aaron can be aware of errors when he does his legacy project."

"Are you proposing a time debt?"

"I guess so—for myself, at least. The time debt of avoiding warning signs."

"Anyone else?" Others rise and offer time debts of ignorance, persistent habits of force, anxiety, and disinterest.

Sarah says, "What happened here is important for Aaron— and for all of us who look ahead to our lifeworks and legacies, and who bear witness to these new consort vows. Let's take an hour of shared contemplation during which we purify the harm of our hell states, and their fixed misperceptions, and the loss that the sisters and their families and all of us have created by our errors."

6

Reggie's Legacy

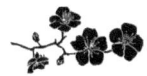

On the first Sunday morning of the lunar month, as the morning fog dampens the skin and clothing of those on stage, Sarah is the one who is having trouble remaining serene and optimistic. Reggie's legacy is the one that Melissa knew very little about—apart from the community vision and formation that Reggie shared during the gathering in 2010. This is the story of the community most likely—she believes—to provide Aaron with the chance to see what they were able to do and what they should have done. This is the day that Sarah hopes will enter into his being and inspire his legacy.

Aaron's thoughts are darker than Sarah realizes. He doubts that he will accept the legacy—not because he does not want to, but because he has not seen a way open. If he does not have a glimmer of an idea today, he will have to delay or perhaps even refuse the legacy at the conclusion of the enactments. This would cause difficulties for everyone. He is relieved when the waiting is over, when Sarah introduces the fourth enactment to an expectant, overflowing crowd and the lights go down.

The lights come up on a meeting of the founders that is already in progress. Colette is saying that she would like to raise a concern. There is some debate as to how to raise a scientific versus a spiritual concern. Reggie, who has been silent, says firmly, "I'd like to hear your concern now."

"I've been noticing my state of being, and how it determines the content of my thoughts. My state is rarely fertile, which means that my thoughts run to the sterile, or the deathly. I'm in a creative generative state—a fertile state—when I anticipate union, or contemplate our third—or imagine a living future. I'd like my resting state to be a fertile one—and I'd like the resting state of the group to be a fertile one, too!"

They all turn to Lisa as she says anxiously, "I don't want us to be in a fertile state all the time. That could destabilize the group."

"That's a fair point," Reggie says in her usual understatement.

"I think that to rest in a fertile state we'd have to learn to uncouple it from arousal—and recouple it when we practice union," Colette says.

Randall says, "I think what Collo is saying is that we should be ready to be creative and respond to situations free of preconceived notions."

Reggie replies abruptly, "Collo said what she meant. What I'd like to know, Collo, is this: has your fertile state been useful in your work?"

"Yes—in marveling at conception and pregnancy, delighting in a newborn, nurturing growth, differentiating treatments, or developing new ideas about fertility. We could probably use it for cultivating and restoring habitat."

"How's your state coming along?" Graeme asks.

"Here," Colette says. "Feel this." She looks at Randall. They unite their gazes, create a strong fertile state, and share it with those in the theater.

"It isn't a pure state," Graeme muses.

"I reckon it could be," Reggie says, "if we allowed it to be different to the states we know, and took time to develop it."

Randall moves to speak. Lisa signals him shyly to wait and says, "Let's hold the question now."

Aaron feels her tension. She is afraid. His care state intensifies automatically.

Randall says, "I'm not ready to hold the question. I've been watching my states, too, and noticing what Melissa calls care and cure states. I use a care state to listen to patients, and a cure state in surgery. I should get to know all three and their consequences before trying to change my baseline."

"This is a fertility community," Reggie points out. "Not a medical one."

Aaron feels their fraught state of interbeing, and says, "Stop!" The actors freeze. The stage lights dim. A spotlight goes up on the stage audience.

Aaron says, "The founders seem to be finding their way to reconciling human time debts through habitat restoration—and creating new debts as they go. Is that what you want us to see?"

"What new debts?"

"Randall and Graeme and Reggie speak freely and fearlessly while the others expect force and experience intimidation. These patterns interfere with brainstorming and disrupt shared inter-being—and could endure as debts."

Parvati replies, "We want you to see the meeting as it was— which means that we will each see it uniquely according to our stances as observers, our habits of observation, and our expectations of the observed. What do others see?"

A hospitality guilder stands and says, "I see the founders expressing a deep-seated fear that few will listen and none will hear."

Dirk stands and says, "I see differences in priming. Some founders are ready to act incisively and others are unclear, undecided, unwilling, or unable."

A fertility guilder stands. "I see them struggling to become aware of the most tenacious time debt in history—the tyranny that leads to secrecy and separation and divides body from being and being from interbeing."

A warrior stands and says, "I see that, too. They are struggling with the subtle consequences of perpetual force, which favors debate over dialogue."

A restoration guilder stands and says, "I see them structuring interbeing with lines of force to the point that they're unfit for restoration and wouldn't have become fit if they hadn't learned to rest in fertile states."

A schooler says, "I see that I underestimated Colette's gifts to us."

An agro guilder stands and says, "I see her moving toward focusing on the bodies of humanity and life instead of on individual humans."

Parvati says, "From this point, the enactment follows the thread of joining being and doing. Let's return to the past now. Go!"

The spotlight goes down and the stage lights go up. After a pause, Graeme says, "Getting back to Lisa's point that we don't know the consequences of resting in a fertile state, and don't want to destabilize our interbeing, we might want to use cure states to face past errors, care states to support the present moment, and fertile states to face the future."

Colette says, "Restoration is present action that corrects past errors and creates a living future. A fertile state joins all three times in support of restoration. It's creative and responsive and can support care and cure as child states."

Reggie says, "I reckon we can use whatever states we need in the moment. The question is, what state to cultivate as the resting state of our group mind. Given we're dedicated to fertility, we should rest in a fertile state, and accept that it'll take us a while to explore and adjust it, and then strengthen it."

Andy says hesitantly, "We talk about fertile transformation, but can't define it. If we rest in fertile states, we'll up our odds of grasping that definition."

Colette looks at Lisa and says, "Let's hold these ideas for a moment."

After a polite pause, during which Andy, Colette and Lisa close their eyes and Reggie, Randall and Graeme look restless, Colette says, "A fertile state might give us a little push. We need a vision, too, something to give us a little pull."

Randall says, "I like the idea of setting something behind us and something in front of us to create the envelope of our doing."

There are several discussions that follow that seem to Aaron to split hairs; he is not sure if he is failing to appreciate the details or if they are losing the thread. He soon suspects that the meandering course of development is what they mean to depict. He makes a mental note to set aside any lingering expectations of linear progress and to expect and to be patient with the confusion and uncertainty that will give way, with persistence, to clarity.

In the next scene, the community has a chance to enjoy the humor inherent in this through Andy, whose earthy virtues Aaron is beginning to appreciate. Andy enters stage left wearing a bush hat, ankle boots, and shorts. He is carrying an armload of two by fours. His movements are angular, abrupt, and sure.

Reggie enters stage right. Upon seeing her, Andy puts down his load and asks, "So what did the builders on Saturna say about our lodge?"

"They like cob houses," she says reluctantly.

He sets down his load. "Let's have it, then."

"In their way of thinking, we've made every possible mistake—degraded the habitat, hired the wrong architect, engaged the wrong contractors."

Andy takes off his hat. "We hired the best available. People who know what they're doing and know how to stay in business."

"By behaving as if we can do without life on earth. It has no cash value—and neither do we. We have to make that right."

"Ah look, it takes time to push the frontier. We'll always be out of date."

"We don't have to be clueless. Take the concrete foundation. It has too low an ash content, and comes from far away, which means we've already spent our energy budget. Even by the tepid standards of the triple bottom line, we pushed the environmental tally way into the red."

"Look, contractors work to regulations, and use a profit structure they trust. They're not going to change for us, and we can't afford to change them."

"Or to win the race to the bottom. The homeless have already taken that cup."

Andy clears his throat by way of objection, then picks up his load with a leery look and walks stage left.

Colette enters stage right, breathless, and asks, "What did they say?"

Andy stops and replies, "They said to stop and dig up the foundation."

"Oh! That's a relief! We knew were going in the wrong direction."

Andy puts down his load and turns stage right as Randall bursts onstage and asks breathlessly, "What did they say?"

Andy says sardonically, "They said we have to build a house of straw, or of sticks, or of bricks."

Randall smiles. "Old thinking can be outside the box."

"And outside the lodge."

Graeme enters stage right with Lisa. They ask in unison, "What happened?"

Andy says, "We're going to have to put the trees back."

Reggie says to Graeme, "Except for the wood we milled, the materials we plan to order are toxic and come from far away. We're set to enable consumptive destruction and poisoning of more than one habitat. Plus, we won't do anything to grow the new economy."

Andy says ironically, "Let's jump in the hole and keep digging. That'll give us the room we need for rainwater catchment and sewage composting."

Graeme says, "If we go with the living building paradigm, we'll be moving straight to sustainability and save effort in the long run."

Lisa says, "We'd save even more effort by moving toward self-sufficiency in animal husbandry as well as gardening."

Andy asks ironically, "You want to house the animals on the first floor?"

"I like the way you think," Lisa says, just as ironically.

More seriously, Andy says, "Look, if we're going to build *our* way, we'll have to come up with specs of our own and recruit mates to throw in with us—share the land as well as the labor."

"No voting rights. The six of us have to work things out first," Reggie says. "Know anyone who needs work?"

"A few good blokes who could use a break—and who might be willing to put up with this mob." The lights go down.

New images come up on the panels. The central panel shows a photo of the partially-constructed lodge with hothouses, garden, and the alder seedlings that mark the theater's beginnings. The panel stage left shows a fabro complex made of old sails and other scavenged materials. The panel stage right shows a yurt camp where the concepto center stands today. The stage lights go up on a thrust stage topped by a long curving pile of soil. Beside the soil lie picks and shovels. Twenty or so seedlings sit on the main stage. Graeme and Randall are carrying seedlings to the thrust stage and placing them at even intervals along the soil.

Randall says pensively, "I'm liking the esoteric practice that you came up with. It's repatterning my actions."

"But?"

"I lose it whenever I start a task. I can think and talk about what I do in a new way, but when I set out to do it, I fall into the old patterns."

Graeme kneels and sits on his heels. "It will take time for your stances and states to harness your priming and to pattern your strategies and skills—and your embodiment of them."

Randall kneels beside him, saying, "I've trained before. I learn best by doing. If I don't get the train in motion now I never will. Walk me through it?"

"I can give it a go." Graeme closes his eyes. After a pause he says, "I'm not ready. When I move, I optimize my movements like a machine. That's from my years as a miner in Western Australia. When I care for life, I try to adjust it the way I would in physiotherapy."

"We don't know how to do this!" Randall exclaims. "In the past I learned by imitation. I developed some new procedures of my own, but they were variations of existing ones. I don't know how to do something that's new to my body—like planting a tree."

"I reckon no one does. It's best to start with what we know."

"I don't know how to entrain a fertile state. I don't think I do any task that moves from priming to stance to state to strategy to skill."

Graeme smiles crookedly. "That's not what I hear."

"We know union."

"You know it better than I do. You can improvise."

"What makes you say that?"

"This is a very small community. We know each other through and through."

"You want me to make love to the seedlings?" Randall laughs. "I can't. I don't feel what moves them. I could bless them. That would at least keep me from controlling the forest—which would be worse than neglecting it."

"I reckon we'll have to learn to feel it. Why don't we try to prime our stance for change, entrain it to a fertile state, and envision a thriving habitat to invite new strategies and skills."

After a pause, Randall smiles and inhales deeply. "Okay. Now what?"

"Let's plant—without losing our state. See how it affects our movements."

Randall stands slowly, eyes still closed. "How about some music?"

"Sing our planting the way indigenous Aussies sing lines across the land?"

"Do you know how?"

"No."

"Then let's sing fertility." Randall clears his throat, inhales deeply, and begins to sing the Song of Songs in Hebrew. Graeme overlays a contrapuntal Tibetan chant. The lights go down.

A voice calls out, "Stop!" The house lights go up. A young fabro guilder stands and says, "The divide between being and doing was empty then, and it's empty now. For all I know, fabro and concepto guilders may be filling it, but I don't entrain fertile states in my work."

A young agro guilder stands and says, "Concepto and restoro hold our mission and we serve them. That isn't what I wanted."

"What did you want?" Aaron asks.

"I wanted my work to go somewhere and mean something. We solve pressing problems and have fun doing it, but we don't develop states or link them with a larger purpose."

A hospitality guilder stands and says, "Sarah holds us together, and we're glad she does because we're doing all we can."

Belatanu stands and says, "We stepped down human transformation to step up fertile restoration of the body of life."

Dirk stands and says, "Warriors make a point of deepening and shifting states to develop doing—and vice versa."

Another warrior guilder stands and says, "But we go on doing what we do. We don't develop new ways of living—and don't try."

Rafa says, "Or you're becoming aware that you're ready to do it."

A hospitality elder stands and says, "We may have set aside modern—and pre-modern—systems, but we're recreating some of the old divisions."

A fabro elder stands and says, "We sync as a community

because we sync with the seasons. If we didn't, we'd see that we're moving ahead separately."

Aaron asks with a keen frown, "You're out of sync with each other?"

Sarah says, "Now that the founders are gone, no one is holding our center or envisioning our future. I hope you will use your perspective as outsiders to discover our errors and give us advice."

"I see your concern better now," Aaron replies.

"So do I!" Rafa adds.

"Go!" Parvati declares. The lights go down.

The lights go up on another meeting of the founders. Aaron is shocked as they begin—abruptly—to argue. Their voices are raised, and Reggie especially is livid. At first, he has trouble grasping what is going on, but soon manages to dial into the substance of the argument and to follow the dialogue.

Reggie is railing, "Melissa should be with John, and both should be here with us! I can't believe you took their repetitive self-punishing thoughts at face value!"

"You're making much too much of this," Graeme objects with a laugh.

"You broke your promise to put aside your special powers and work with us as equals! You imposed your will on all of us—and at the expense of the very people who made it possible for us to do the work we're doing! The very people who should be here to give us the bandwidth we need!"

Colette says calmly, "Tell us what happened."

After a tense pause, Reggie inhales raggedly and tells Colette, "Graeme exercised his special powers to rearrange Melissa's life without her knowledge or consent—and without talking it over with you or Randall."

Colette asks incredulously, "Graeme, did you break into their minds?"

"They didn't know, and I only gave them what they wanted."

"You barely know them. How could you possibly guess what they wanted?"

Andy says, "He supported marriage vows."

Lisa says, "He helped all of us save face."

Colette asks Andy and Lisa, "Did he mention this to you before taking unilateral action? Or ask for your consent?"

Andy sighs and looks at Lisa. They shake their heads reluctantly.

Reggie says to Graeme, "I made it clear that I wanted no part of guru yoga and you promised to give up hierarchy—and every kind of force."

Graeme replies darkly, "I worked long and hard for my powers. I'm not going to give them up. I won't violate my original vows, either, or let my practices lapse, or answer to anyone who's beneath me in my lineage."

"What did you do?" Randall asks ominously.

Reggie replies, "He came between Melissa and John."

Randall looks at Colette in dismay. She nods grimly.

"Can you undo it?" Randall asks.

"Not without using special powers."

"We have to find a way to talk with them about it," Randall says to Colette.

"We might lose Melissa. You know her conscience. It's harsh, and punitive."

Reggie hisses. "You violated my trust and my body. I renounce you as my consort!" She turns and exits stage right.

Colette hesitates, and then says, "We can't cooperate with

nature if we can't cooperate with each other, and we can't cooperate with each other through ego—or stealth." She backs away and then turns and runs after Reggie, exiting stage right.

Aaron is shocked. He looks at Rafa, and sees she is also shocked. The founders expected Melissa and John to come here and join them in their work. The founders had chosen them as founders—all but Graeme, who had broken into her mind, changed the course of her life, and spoiled her happiness. A stranger's presumptuous interference had changed the course of Aaron's life. Aaron looks at John, who seems calm. Perhaps he had heard this in the lead up to the enactments.

Randall looks at Graeme incredulously. "I can't believe your arrogance. Andy and Lisa have stuck to their vows with great difficulty, and I applaud them, but not everyone does that for the best. Melissa and John were finally ready to admit that everyone would be better off if they each divorced and then married one another. You can't impose your will as if it were the right thing to do—especially when you don't know them. Eavesdropping for a few days can't tell you what years of knowing them has revealed to us. Melissa's devotion to Dan is self-punishment, not love, and Dan imagines that he isn't abusive because he has a persecution complex. John spent too much time at work to be a part of his family. They were all about to change for the better."

Andy says, "They made vows and they're keeping them. They'll come right."

Randall adds, "Melissa and John have been consorts since they were teens. Their marriage vows were false from the start. Their work wasn't. They could have been happy with us and catalyzed works of genius here."

Graeme says. "Life transforms as one being, and in its own time. No one person or consort couple can speed it up or slow it down."

Andy looks at Randall, and asks Graeme, "Then what are we all doing here? And what were you doing interfering?"

Randall says, "It looks like we won't be doing anything." He turns away and exits stage right.

Graeme looks uneasily after Randall as Andy and Lisa exit center stage under the image of the main door. The lights go down. "Stop!" calls a bass voice. The house lights go up.

A concepto elder stands and says, "I don't remember hearing of any formative crisis, and I'm not sure what to take away from this aspect of the enactment. This seems like a cautionary tale that is key now, when Sarah is nearing the end of her years and Aaron's legacy is poised to change our patterns. I'd like to know what you'd like us to learn from this, and what others think of it."

A restoration elder stands and says, "Randall told me that the founders relied on Reggie's New Direction practice at the first, which began with forming a vision based on the ultimate intention and priming based on residual hell states. She developed it for use in her work as a winemaker, so she could have used it for the retreat, but I see no signs of it, and wonder if they didn't use it or if Graeme violated it."

Parvati replies, "We chose to show the confusion during the first scene only. They did use the New Direction practice and it was—for our purposes—uneventful, whereas Randall's comment on something behind and something ahead shaped the entrainment process that you described and that we still use to join being and doing."

"Thanks for the clarification."

A concepto initiate stands and says, "I'm shocked that Graeme behaved the way he did. Do you think they wanted to conceal his breach of ethics for fear that students would hear of it and stay away?"

Doug says, "I think they were ashamed. I know they were."

Parvati says, "I would say that they felt intense regret, and used the incident to motivate the development of new practices for grounding and patterning their work in life and time."

A warrior guilder stands and says, "They may have used an early version of our practice of completion. In that practice, you take action to correct an error and then think and speak of it no more."

Aaron says, "Wait a minute—this sounds like self-governance. Are you saying that you rely on your esoteric practices for self-governance?"

Sarah says, "Not exactly. We use evolving narratives as means for entraining states and strategies to our shared purpose after grounding all of us in shared time and each of us in personal time."

Rafa asks, puzzled, "Your grounding in time is your governance?"

Parvati says, "Not exactly. Sarah, as storykeeper, coordinates the interactive formation of our shared narrative on a daily basis, and steps in where habit fails. We structure our personal narrative around our vocations."

Aaron's view of their problem clicks into place. "You run on habit?"

A warrior guilder says, "We sustain subtle—and not so subtle—social processes that ground us in time and place that you should include in your thinking as you review our governance."

Aaron shakes his head in disbelief, and says with an ironic laugh, "I'm glad you got around to mentioning it."

Parvati laughs and says, "We didn't want it to color your view of our history."

"Please continue. I'll have to listen and come back with questions later. I may have been looking without seeing."

Oke Ten stands and says, "We can see that it's time to change our grounding in life in time, and don't want to change it lightly because it can lead to instabilities."

After a polite pause, another older warrior stands and says, "I imagine that the founders concealed this error as a way of allowing Graeme to work with his lineage to create new vows so that he could work on an equal basis with the founders."

Parvati says, "This scene and our warriors' remarks remind us that to change at a deep level, we must change along with everyone connected to us."

Aaron says patiently, "You do realize that's impossible."

"In a living system, it's inevitable." Sarah interjects. "You can anticipate and prepare for a singularity, but precipitating it can injure shared—and individual interbeing."

Parvati says to Aaron, "The important thing is to let go of the past and lead the future."

"To remove obstacles to movement?" he asks sharply.

"Yes."

Doug says, "Like your mom and John did in their medical work."

Rafa asks, "What was that practice the founders were using— the one Reggie developed in Australia?"

"The New Direction practice patterned transformative self-governance as a process of commitment, consensus, co-transformation and continuation."

The elder warrior guilder adds, "We entrained those steps with restorative stances and fertile states, and added strategies and skills, but it was never robust. We had to share our basic practices and narrative as often, and as unobtrusively, as we could."

Aaron says, "Less structure would favor deeper change."

"And come with more risk."

"Is it inherent and unavoidable risk, perhaps?"

John says, "Stepwise change is safer. Melissa thought they were already changing too much too fast, and might fall apart."

Oke Ten replies, "We were about to retire the old practices because they seem to hold us back. Perhaps we should keep them for times like this, when change could destabilize our ground."

"For now, at least," Parvati says. "This is not the time to limit our possibilities—or to lose our grounding."

Sarah says, "I'd like to make one more point about the scene by way of apology for Graeme. The founders were just learning to work with time. Graeme's grounding was deepest, and his transition was slowest and most difficult. In other words, he had become deeper at the cost of becoming narrower."

Parvati says, "Thank you. Let's move on now to the next and final scene of this last enactment, which may address some of your remarks. Go!" The lights go down.

A panoramic image comes up on the panels behind the stage that shows a sloop moored in Burrard Inlet. In the foreground is Stanley Park; in the background is Grouse Mountain. On the thrust stage sits the ruin of an old boat deck. Reggie is leaning beside the helm and Colette is seated on a bench.

Colette asks, "What did we do wrong?"

Reggie shakes her head, "What I did wrong was to take

Graeme's word as his bond. I knew when we first met that he didn't feel bound to friends or family—or even to me, but I thought he'd got past that. I never thought he'd be a Nosey Parker, or interfere so casually."

"Their thoughts must have annoyed him."

Reggie grunts and puts her hands over her face. After a pause, she says, "It's hard for me to see this right now, but I think he wanted to be useful to them. I think that part of it was sincere." She folds her arms.

Colette says, "From what I could tell, Melissa was in pain. I wonder why he didn't ease her pain instead of changing the course of her life!"

"That's what's upsetting me most. His judgment is terrible outside of a very narrow set of circumstances. And he doesn't see it! He can't always handle himself—and can't tell when he can't. How can I trust him?"

"Are you sure you're ready to talk about what to do next? Maybe you need some time to reflect—and maybe he'll repent, and reconcile with us."

"I can't count on him."

"We're all going to make mistakes, and some of them will be serious. We have to bounce back from this or give up, and it's way too early to give up."

"And we can't. I've been sitting with the looming extinction, and consulting with my contacts in France who look at agronomy from the standpoint of field biology. Things are dire. We can't quit—but we may have to go on without Graeme. I may have to look for a new consort who knows how to handle himself in this kind of situation."

"Do you have someone in mind?"

"No. No one who's willing or able to cross the divide between being and doing what needs doing in the world. The potential consorts I know renounce life, and they have no strategies or skills—which means they rely on deception for a living."

"Deception?"

"Look, there's a reason I'm a solo tantrika. I follow Western forms of equality, transparency, and responsibility."

"You wouldn't want to lose that."

Reggie sighs. "Thanks for the support. I'm so glad you came with me. I'm used to handling things on my own, and I cherish solitude, but I never want to work alone again. That's another reason I blew up. You and Randall and Andy and Lisa mean more to me than family, and Graeme did too—until now. It's frightening. We can work all our lives to create and continue our integrity—inside and out—and lose it all in a minute."

"Let's not create a self-fulfilling prophecy. Let's use this to become more resilient. But how?"

Reggie groans and answers, "What I learned in my work is that we need to develop—at the very least—practices that pattern commitment, consensus-as-transformation, and continuation. In other words, we have to agree on what we're going to do and how we're going to be effective. To do that, we have to commit, and carry on."

"This raises the issue of force. We're all moderns—or pre-moderns, I guess—and we all have force in us. It's practically our ground. Graeme is too quick to use it—and to use it unilaterally. You can't work with nature that way. It's essential to allow life on earth to lead, and then to work with it, to cooperate and interact with it, and to move ahead as one. That's what agronomy brought to society and it's still in us—even when we lose our ties to nature, we retain the capacity to cooperate with it."

"We've been enjoying the fruits of it—until now."

"We have to build on that—and take it into our fertility work. Every habitat is human-modified by now—if it survives. The question is, do we need force to cure nature or do we go with pure fertile, creative cooperation?"

"I'm not fond of meeting bears. You can't be in the wild without taking responsibility for being prey as well as predator. We'll have to use force if we're to protect our lives. We're not ready to lay down with the lion."

"We don't live in Alaska. We don't need to carry a shotgun, or rifle."

"True."

"For now, we need to clear ourselves of force, and to rely on love."

"Are you climbing up on the cross?" Reggie asks with a laugh.

"No. I'm looking at Graeme from the standpoint of non-violence and I can tell you from personal experience that he can't tell a mind rape from a quick chat."

"He violated your mind?"

"Yes, before. I asked him to never do it again, but he seems to think that he has gone beyond right and wrong. He's living in Orwell's *Animal Farm*, where some of us are more equal than others. I don't think he comprehends consensus."

"I see. You can't have consensus when you seek status—or power."

"Exactly. Assent and consent and consensus are subject to influence. We have to be sure they're free and clear and conscientious in our case. Quakers struggled with it and some have done it, which means that we can do it."

Reggie hugs herself. "I know I put us here, but I feel trapped. Trapped on the deck of this boat, trapped with a consort I'm struggling to respect, trapped on an island that's—well, insular—and trapped in a country that doesn't know it's a set of habitats."

"I have an idea," Colette says. "In peacemaking, we talk of dialogue and reconciliation. We could take those practices and adapt them to our work. The Abrahamic creeds talk of forgiving debts. Melissa's talked about measuring and paying our debts in time—like the time it would take to make amends or to repent. Graeme could own his mistakes and formulate them as debts of time—time debts. He could return life in time to the state or condition it would have been in if he hadn't made the mistake."

"How would you measure it?"

"Conscientiously, in the body. We can all feel when we've done wrong, and when we've made it right."

"According to our views—which may be off."

"We can't do it if we don't try. And it's our ultimate purpose. We have to work together the way we work with nature."

Reggie pauses. "Good point."

"What I have to bring to this is the lessons of the radical reformation. We have no clergy here—and Graeme's problems are clerical. Lollards started the theological processes that Quakers extended in order to meet God without an intermediary."

"Oh, God, you're right," Reggie declares. "We're not practicing what we preach."

"We're not going deep enough—Graeme is probably showing what all of us are doing deep down, in some way."

"I wish we could do it with John and Melissa."

"I would have liked things to turn out differently, but it may be for the best. And we have to give Graeme credit for planting all those trees."

"With Randall. Their egos match well—too well."

"I agree," Colette says. "Randall's a surgeon, and I love him for it, and I want him to continue with it, but he's going to have to find a way to shift into a different gear when he's doing fertility work."

"As opposed to infertility work."

"Right."

"Is that why you suggested a fertile state as the baseline?"

"Yes. I have to compensate for his state and I don't want to spend my energy on that."

"We need a vision."

"What about the one you shared when Missy was here?"

"It's time to make it clearer—and more interactive. It has to support us forming new practices that repattern our lives as we gain experience."

"Are we taking on too much?"

"We have to change the way we change, and we have to change it continually."

"That's what you and Graeme took as your third. It's a worthy task, and the rest of us should help, but only you and he can work this out. What were you saying about responsibility?" Colette asks shyly.

Reggie snorts, "I reckon I don't like it."

The lights go down.

Aaron realizes, with a dizzying telescoping of time, that the founders were different rather than gifted, wise rather than brilliant. He can see now that his mother was the hidden visionary and Reggie the teacher who caressed, castigated, and cajoled her listeners to disillusion them of the sterile modern promise of money and status. It was she who revealed the too-familiar elisions and compromises of mind they had made and rationalized and forgotten. It was she who turned idea into impact.

It is his turn now to do what the founders did then—to discern or devise a way to catalyze the continuing metamorphosis of this community. Before, he expected to accept the legacy out of duty; now he feels as if his whole body is pressed against the glass of a door that he must push open to move into the future. He longs for this. This is his chance to offset his errors, mischances, and mislaid plans with grounded faith, reasonable hope, and fertile generation.

In his body, the curses of destruction intermingle with the blessings of restoration. He took the year zero here—the year the community formed—as the hinge of human history, but realizes now that time is long and reckoned continuously in each life. The hinge is behind him, with him, ahead of him. Past, present, and future live in him as an ongoing evolution that favors continuation.

Growing up with illness in the home taught him to choose life by nurturing virtues like steadfastness, tenaciousness, and persistence. Life has been preparing him to accept that only the Torah of Life in Time can guide him—the Torah of unending creation. The future of life is not certain—however much he might wish otherwise. He, too, must go forth and multiply, but he will multiply the self-patterning for change that he saw today in the enactment. Their self-governance, having let go of the ritual combat of legal debate, has become cryptic. There is little shared God-wrestling, and less deep, non-consensual dialogue. The discordant fire of cure has died down to embers.

7

Entanglement

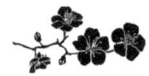

Rafa opens the screen door and enters the dining room of the main lodge, where she sees that almost all the residents and guests have taken off the formal clothes of their vocations and adorned themselves in elaborate costumes, some of which reveal intricate body paintings in henna or broad brush paintings in pigmented, scented body oils or creams. Her first impulse is to laugh. She sees in them the obsessive need for attention or social ascendancy that she had witnessed in the forlorn souls that haunted the streets of Denver. She soon realizes, though, that she is perceiving it wrongly, and the urge to laugh grows still. The adornment is expressing something of the vibrant zest that fills the room. She lets it expand her being and fuel her becoming.

She presses into the crowd as into a part of the body of humanity that feels fathomless and limitless. She senses joy, delight, triumph, parental love, and mysterious states that she can recognize, but cannot name. She realizes with a jolt that they are out of sync. She has never detected this before. In the whole of her life, every gathering she has attended began with people coming together in states that were fragmented or complex or fraught. Here, almost every individual sustains a state that is deep and constant and perfectly integrative of a myriad of personal processes. The shared state in the room is one of intense exuberant accord marked by dysrhythmic clashes that trigger intervals of stillness or foreboding. The body of the community seems to resemble a precessing gyroscope that is pitched to go out of balance. She feels what is worrying Sarah and grasps the task ahead of *Tío*. Rafa is glad that it does not fall to her. She looks for Yukie, but does not see her or anyone else she knows.

After a time, an agro guilder by the name of Damian enters and introduces himself to her as having lineal roots among the Saami people. He explains that this is north of Rafa's roots— through Melissa—in the Ätran watershed of old Sweden. For his initiation project, Damian joined a restoration team above the Arctic Circle so as to revisit his roots. He learned to live with the wild, and to make a new kind of cheese from reindeer milk and berries. Rafa recognizes Damian's costume from images she has seen while passing through the residential part of the lodge.

"I think I passed by the door of your cell. Your costume is like the pictures on one of the doors."

"Yes! This lei is for Saint Damien of Molokai; this is like the robe of Saint Damien shown in an old icon of the Arabic doctor twins—that's for you and your family—and this body painting is of the Hippocratic tree on Kos—also in honor of your family— and the headdress is for the shaman who mentored me in reindeer care, and the bark cloth is for people who cared for forest before the white and gray tides flooded the land with the rest of us."

"White and gray tides?"

"The immigrations after 1491—people and rats."

"What are those tatts?"

"These are for my commitments. This is for my habitat—I'm littoral, like Yukie—and this is the agro tatt, and this one is for my declaration of simple-same, and these are for my one-and three-year consortships."

"I thought it was just a costume."

"It is. Appearance is always a costume, and always tells a story."

"I dress to hide my story," she smiles.

"Don't look now, mate, but your story's showing," Damian says with a wink.

Rafa tries to read Damian's state and senses that it is akin to anticipation. After a pause, she says, "I'll have to read it and maybe revise it."

"You're uncommitted. Wear and share. What do you want to share?"

"Confusion?"

"You're wearing it, mate." He laughs.

As she moves on to try to find Yukie, Rafa realizes that she cannot enjoy the wild colors, textures, patterns, and meanings that surround her. She cannot read the crowd. She has taken her manner of dress and that of John, Doug, *Tío*, and the visitors as the normal dress that sets off all the rest. She closes her eyes and feels their states of being flooding her core. It is overwhelming. She hurries out into the cold night and heads toward the forest.

When she reaches a red cedar, which she can barely see in the dim light from the dining room windows, she leans against its trunk. As she recovers, Rafa realizes that she has been drawing on the forest since the day of her arrival. While this part of the body of humanity could crush her core, this part of the body of life expands it. She loves the forest. She is enchanted with it, in love with it. If she did not know about shakedown or empties, she would want to partner it. She must grow stronger first. In the meantime, she can nurture—perhaps mother—the forest.

Rafa glimpses her future: she will become a habitat restorer. She will make and trade clinics to catalyze restoration of the forest. There is nothing for it. She was born to be a restorer and is already becoming one. She inherited this destiny from her doctor ancestors who discovered that they could best treat individual humans in the context of the bodies of humanity and of life. She already craves this lifework as she craves water when thirsty, or food when hungry, or exercise when sitting. But she cannot do it here; she must do it in a place or places where life is struggling. Her clinics must start with the soil; perhaps they will use domes. She cannot tell. The only thing she can tell is that she will not be here long, and will not end her days here.

Rafa feels *Tío* standing behind her. She is not sure how she knows who it is before she hears his kind voice. She realizes that she loves him intensely. No wonder Parvati is gravitating toward *Tío* like the earth to the sun.

"Come with us," *Tío* says soothingly. "The others are ready to hold us."

Rafa's throat thickens. She can feel her mother's love awakening inside her, something she has not felt since her arrival. She nods and follows her uncle around to the far side of the dining room and inside. They ascend a moveable stair to mount a high platform made of tables. She goes to stand beside Yukie, scanning the crowd and wondering what kind of costume she should wear. She knows that she belongs now, and always will.

Sarah faces the crowd in the dining room, which extends outside through every doorway, and says brightly, "It's time to hear from Aaron, and to pause for thanks and blessings. How did you find the enactments?"

Rafa is amazed at Sarah's energy. She has more vitality than

John, who is leaning on Gina, or Doug, who is too stubborn to lean on Sarah, whom he watches with a skeptical eye. Rafa smiles when Aaron fails to note that Sarah is speaking to him. Yuki takes his arm, and he comes out of his reverie with a start to scan the crowd. "Well," he says, looking into her smiling eyes, "that's a big question."

Rafa's heart sinks. She has seen *Tío* in communicator mode. He can temporize, deflect, and make nice without saying anything meaningful. As Rafa surveys the crowd, she can see that she might do the same if she could. The expressions of anticipation could dry up a well-rehearsed expert performer with classical lines to remember.

Tío braces himself and says openly, "I've taken them in, but it will be a long time before I reconcile them with my early memories. I can say now that I am privileged to have seen this transmission; challenged by the thought that you put into it; amazed to have taken an actress for an incarnation of my mother," he says with a light laugh, "and daunted by the task of comprehending it all and making good on it. Since it's time for thanks, I can also express my dumbfounded gratitude to your kindred and connections—most especially Mom's friends of nearly eighty years; to your highly attuned knowledge keeper, Parvati; and to the performance and fabro guilders who took us back in time to see, own, and interact with our history. I'll be scratching my head and thinking how to embody it."

"Thanks for letting me to get to know her all over again," Doug says.

"Thank you for letting us spend time with her," John says, his voice breaking.

"I have something to say to the cast!" Doug exclaims

facetiously. "Remember that you've been monumental versions of people who were small and ordinary and didn't inspire us until after the fact. So leave your role onstage. You're small and ordinary enough already."

The performance guilders laugh under their breath and shake their heads.

Sarah says, "Fortunately, you all know what went as planned and what didn't. We'll have to let Doug guess at what we saw from the stage, and backstage."

Björn lifts Parvati onto the platform between Rafa and Yukie and jumps up to join them, mic in hand. He gives it to Sarah. Yukie hands Björn two huge folios that she has been holding.

Sarah continues, as if announcing welcome news, "Tonight's enactment marks the completion of Aaron's legacy transmission!"

Björn leads the crowd in a cheer by bellowing, "Hurrah! Hurrah! Hurrah!"

Sarah resumes, her weary eyes lit by a satisfied smile. "Aaron, we have been privileged to share these stories with you. Now, for—"

"Wait!" Björn growls. "I reckon you've seen that Melissa was key in Randall's thinking. She was behind a lot of what we are—and what we do. It's time to recognize that she was one of our founders! If you agree, chant with me: Melissa! Melissa! Melissa! Melissa! Melissa!"

A few join him, and then a few more, and then a hundred, and then almost everyone present.

Björn raises his arms for quiet and says, "Let's take a vote!"

"Vote! Vote! Vote!" chants the crowd, intensifying the energy in the room.

"Now?" Björn shouts.

"Now! Now! Now!" they chant with increasing speed.

Björn cups his hands around his mouth and booms, "All in favor of adding Melissa to the list of founders, say Aye!"

"Aye! Aye! Aye!"

"All against say Nay."

Parvati hears a smattering of voices saying, "Nay."

Björn shouts, "The Ayes have it! Recognizing a lost founder will remind us that we're only just beginning to make good on all our blessings!"

Björn turns and winks at Sarah, who puts her hand on her heart in gratitude.

Sarah continues. "Björn will now give you these beautifully illustrated volumes that record the legacy enactment. The fabro guild prepared them for you to commemorate this transmission."

Aaron smiles broadly, takes the folios, and thanks her.

"As you know," Sarah says with a laugh that betrays anxiety, "we are all wondering whether you have decided to accept your legacy and prepare for a three-month legacy retreat."

Sarah hands Aaron the microphone. The hall falls silent. Aaron says, "Thank you all for sharing your amazing history, and for giving me this chance to continue the work that I witnessed as a young man, and that continues to be so intimately connected with my family. This has been a profound and life-changing experience for me and Rafa. You have charged us with new purpose and meaning.

"I can tell you right now that I accept the legacy and look forward to a three-month retreat during which to contemplate it." Rafa sees relief on Sarah's face, and is relieved herself to see that *Tío* is happy. The community whoops and applauds; many members dance. When the crowd finally grows quiet again, he continues, "I promise to do all that I can to rise to the challenge you have set! Thank you for the opportunity presented by high expectations and for your understanding that I will do my best.

"Looking back on each enactment, we can see one message that stands out. The first encourages us to accept what we don't know and to engage the unknown; the second shows us that we can get to the root of a problem and create unprecedented solutions; the third reminds us that we have to, and can, make much use of chance and circumstance to change deeply; and the fourth challenges us to fail and to open to darkness in order to seek and appreciate light. All that we have to do now is to define the problem and create a solution," he jokes.

"And now, before we go, I would like to ask you to reconcile one more time debt. That debt is to John, who deserves a place with my mother and your other founders. I ask you now to take a minute to consider recognizing him as a founder and a consort of my mother, and to join his family memorial with ours."

Aaron turns to John, who is sitting sadly on a chair set against the west wall next to Gina. Aaron begins applauding. He looks out over the audience and gestures to invite them to applaud John with him. Björn jumps down, goes to retrieve John, and places him between Sarah and Aaron on the platform. Aaron takes John's hand and raises it.

Dirk begins the chant, "John, John, John, John ... "

The chant spreads and grows louder. Sarah and Parvati are taken unawares. Björn hops up on the platform again and bellows, "Will someone make the motion to include John in the group of founders?"

"I will!" shouts Doug.

Sarah recovers and laughs. "Thank you, Doug. An initiated member?"

"I will," says Parvati.

"I second the motion," says the performance guilder who played Randall in middle age. "This will bring us closer to syncing with Aaron and Rafa."

"Hear, hear!" says Björn.

"All in favor?" asks Sarah.

A roar of ayes rises and echoes from the ceiling. When the voices and applause die away, John takes the microphone, rises to full height, regards the crowd and says, "It's been a long time since I received an award, and none has ever meant more to me than this. I thank you in memory of my beloved, and in the name of every member of her family and mine."

Rafa climbs up on a chair to get a better view of the down-stairs dance room. Outside, in the hallway at the bottom of the stairs, she chose wooden shoes from a huge store of them stashed in cubbies like those in the schoolroom. From the entry she saw a sea of people, and heard the clomping of countless pairs of clogs; from the chair, she can see the room itself. As Yukie explained, it is a long box with a geothermal ceiling that absorbs heat, bioluminescent glass walls that shimmer with green and blue algae that turn heat into iridescent patterns, and a wooden floor covered with thick bark cloths that transfers energy from the dancers' impacts to the lodge's battery array. At the far end of the room is the band that is setting the rhythm: a modified Latin percussion set with a gourd rattle; a single huge taiko drum; a box drum; and a wailing violin. These are setting the pace of the dance, to which the clogs are synchronizing. The dancers are side-by-side and bent at the hips, their torsos parallel to the floor, their arms over their neighbor's backs. They form one sinuous line that describes the seven petals of a flower, the center of which is beginning to fill with those who have finished dancing.

The idea is to release useless burdens like time debts that have been paid or that belong to others, as well as the trivial or useless undigested debts that are stuck in the solar plexus or that have not yet reached it. What debts remain may be useful as priming for initiation, vocation, or legacy.

Rafa has no experience with priming her body, and finds herself with no idea what to release. Yukie has said not to worry, that Rafa's body will release only what it does not need and that the rest of her debts will be transformed into priming as experience allows. Rafa is still reluctant to join in, partly because some of the dancers are retching unpleasantly—but the dancers in the center look so relieved that she resolves to try. Yukie told Rafa that she can drum out her burdens by doing the steps, but that she must first learn to sense and to support this personal, inward process. Fortunately, her work with Belatanu has given her a feel for this—but now she has to figure out the moves.

The steps appear simple; each dancer leaps leftward with the left foot, brings the right foot in and jumps on it, and then stomps on the left and then the right. As dancers enter the center, the line shortens and they move farther with the first step. Rafa tries small steps on the chair seat and finds she catches on quickly. Because the sinuous line is already formed and moving, she will only need to find a way in and follow along.

Rafa spots Belatanu and Damian in the corner nearest her, carrying on a conversation by shouting into each other's ears. Damian keeps glancing at her; perhaps he is curious, or perhaps Belatanu is talking about her. She jumps down and clomps clumsily toward them, her mouth full of questions. She smiles at them both and then goes to Belatanu's other ear to ask, "What do those symbols mean—the ones on the floor cloth?"

"Those symbolize useless burdens and their release in dance," Bel says.

"Undigested experiences, unprocessed memories, maladaptive habits—anything that traps or wastes energy and that you want to release as waste," Damian shouts.

"Are they—are the dancers going to toss their dinner?"

Bel laughs. "Only the undigested experiences that they feel in their sun centers and that they don't want. They're retching to invite those to leave body and being."

"Does that work?"

"I've managed it once or twice. The best thing is that the dance patterns a process of putting out harm. So even when it doesn't work here, it works in your life."

"How do you get in?"

Belatanu holds out his hand. She takes it. His energy enters her palm and surrounds her like a tender embrace. Rafa gasps. She does not want to drum him out; she wants to snuggle up and join now, and for as long as it feels like this.

"Are you all right?" he asks, puzzled.

Rafa realizes that she is staring at him, stupefied. She laughs and nods. He does not appear to share her experience. Setting that aside, she looks to lose herself in the dance.

"I'm ready to get sweaty," she jokes.

Belatanu smiles and leads her to the moving apex of the nearest petal. He puts his arm around her waist and guides hers under his and around his waist. She feels like an elf beside a colossus. He bends forward at the hips and enters the line; she does her best to keep up. It is at first much harder to orient and to hold the rhythm than she expected. She leans on Belatanu and on the girl on her other side to steady herself, and then for physical support.

Rafa suddenly realizes why there are so few older people at the dance: it is physically demanding, and requires a unique form of fitness. The posture is the greatest challenge, and watching the symbols pass without resting her eyes on any is disorienting and dizzying. It takes her several minutes to follow along without making mistakes, and much longer—how long, she is not sure—to move easily with her hips and knees bent and her eyes first on one symbol and then the next.

As the drumming of her feet becomes second nature, she becomes aware that her state is fraught and her mind filled with angry and then sad thoughts. She skips over the horror of her last years in Denver and lands on the anger she has felt at her father's neglect. She tries to feel it in the hollow of her stomach, beneath her ribs, but cannot. Perhaps it is too soon. Rafa then tries to focus on memories of the enactments, but her wariness and dislike of her grandmother and her grandmother's generation are gone. Her thoughts return again and again to her father, and her feelings to a familiar but loathsome mix of rage and want and love; this, it seems, is the burden that is ready for release. She is aware that there may be others soon; she senses them entangled with her stance towards her father.

The burden she encounters is not the litany of complaints and laments that she expected. It is like a tangled nest of eels, some electric; they seem to sting or to slither into shadowy depths. She cannot untangle them at will, nor control the lash and whiplash of sting and punishment, blow and counter blow, transgression and repentance. She begins to sob, and then to cough, and finally to collect what is ready into her sun center and to dry-retch it out of her body.

Rafa relaxes into the arms around her back. The music and the scrolling stomping sweep her away. The dance accelerates. She forgets everything other than coughing up the past and keeping time. As the dance becomes frenetic, more and more dancers step to the center. Finally, the drumbeat ends—but its rhythm continues beating in her bones. She has reached the end of her first cathartic dance. Her body is numb. She moves to the center, exhausted and relieved, and joins in shouting "Life!" She has taken a first giant step toward peace.

Belatanu moves to the center with her. He looks relaxed and joyful as he raises his arms and chest to the ceiling, closes his eyes, and mutters words of gratitude. When the cluster at the center disperses toward the water fountains in the corners or in the vestibule, Belatanu takes her hand again and says, "I think I felt your state more than mine."

"Do you want to go somewhere and ... talk?"

"After the drumming in. I think you'll like it. We can leave early if you like."

"Bueno."

"What does that mean?"

"Good, agreed."

"Did you think of the enactments?"

"No. I thought of my dad. But now ... behind his misery and the faults he imprinted on me, I may find ... something of Grandma, something he passed on to me in spite of himself ... maybe her ability to learn from life, and to find her way ... something of independence and conscience."

Belatanu frowns skeptically.

"Maybe I'm imagining it."

"Maybe ... or maybe the enactment is resonating with you in ways that we didn't expect—which would be great. That's how enactments are. They reveal things we don't—or can't—anticipate."

"Wow. I see what Dirk meant," Rafa says.

"What did he say?"

"He implied that I should let things take their course. But I wish ... I wish I could reach out and take Grandma's perspective, or her ability to read people."

"You wouldn't see those things in her if they weren't in you already."

Rafa sighs and replies incredulously, "That's so ... corroborating ... synergizing."

He smiles pleasure and delight. "That's syncing."

Rafa's mouth opens in amazed recognition as the music begins again. This time, there is no pattern, and the music is salsa-bouncy and invigorating. The dancers keep time by leaping up and down. They move in unison, pushing off and landing with a massive crash that pushes the floor downwards. At first, they leave the balls of their feet on the ground; as the music grows louder and faster, their feet leave the floor. Gradually, they lift higher and higher until they are leaping as high as their shoulders. Rafa contents herself with a hop that she can sustain.

She feels as if her body is an old pot and she is pounding out its dents. It is not long before she feels free of resentments and is jumping in a sea of joy.

While the younger members of the community attend the drumming rites, Sarah leads a small group to the music room on the second floor of the north wing of the lodge. Aaron is surprised to find that the room is windowless and has side and back walls covered by sheer panels of cinnabar silk that offer veiled glimpses of thick cork tiles. A row of high Ottomans stands along the back wall. In the corner beyond them stands a tall cabinet with many niches, drawers, and shelves. Beside it sit stacks of folded sheepskins and baskets of colorful coverlets and blankets.

Each element of the room is alluring; the far wall rivets him. Its luminous blank is like a window into a mysterious fog that promises movement and enchantment. He pulls his eyes away to scan the room and discovers a glass and metal table facing the luminous wall. On top of it stands a fine-grained, lacquered wood frame strung with a delicate mesh made of golden wires and inset with coin-like disks. Below the table hangs a lidded box covered with knobs and gauges. A high cushion is tucked beneath the box.

Doug sits on the nearest cushion at the back, his forearms resting on his knees. Aaron and Parvati take nearby cushions. Gina sits beside Parvati. Sarah approaches the table and pulls out its cushion and fold out and props up a shelf on the right. Then she pulls out a flexible tube and sets it into the lid of the box. She places the box on the shelf, turns a knob and pushes a button. John sits on the high cushion and begins to move his hands over the wire mesh. It is an instrument, and he is tuning it.

A series of images appears on the luminous wall. Aaron recognizes some of them as photos from the enactment; all feature his mother in various times and places. Some show her alone in the wilderness, some indoors with friends, and most with family at home or in far-flung places. Her past rushes by, pulling his with it. He sees his life as a blur of birthday parties; of childhood models of sailing ships; of books, scriptures, and sagas read aloud; and of schooldays and family journeys. The best are over in a flash, and give way to reminders of his long confinement in the comm tower and his parents' institutionalization in their clinic. How little he has lived before now!

"Are you all right? Parvati asks with concern.

Aaron stretches his shirt collar and smiles bravely. "Time is contracting. It's too much, too fast."

"Does seeing the sweep of your life prepare you to take chances?"

"Too late for that!" he exclaims with a trace of bitterness.

Parvati's face contracts, and her fertile state expands to encompass his body. She sighs, recovers, and says teasingly, "A terrible excuse! I would never accept it from a schooler, and no legatee can resist life's greatest adventure."

He laughs. "I ... I've never been one for surprises."

"Surprises are singularities that reveal life's hidden trajectory."

"That sounds like something Mom would say," Aaron remarks.

"That's something John says."

"Ah."

"You're wary of him?"

"I'm challenged by having missed so much of my life. Grateful to see some of that, but non-plussed."

"We're all tired now."

"And how," Doug seconds cantankerously.

Aaron inhales and rallies as all three watch Sarah pull a jar of gel from the box, and then one at a time pull the metal disks from the laquered frame, dab them with gel, and place them on the front and sides of John's body. As she does this, she explains,

"Randall and Graeme helped to develop this instrument—as did John—and called it the composer. The idea was to express the player's state of being as a soundscape. It registers breathing, heartbeat, heat, pulses, blood flows, electrical currents, magnetic fields, and so on. Because John is a musician, he can improvise structured melodies on top of the soundscape. Tonight, he'll play the electronic sax and bass as well as the palmboard. Usually he generates sound and images, but tonight images will inspire his playing."

Sarah puts her hand on John's shoulder. "Will you play Melissa now?"

John nods, then mutters as if he is speaking to the images. Sarah restarts the slideshow, this time in chronological order, beginning with images of Melissa's early life. John grips the edge of the table as if wrestling with unseen angels. The sound is unfocused and, Aaron feels, anticipatory. When the images reach her college years, John puts his lips and tongue on the flexible tube as he adjusts it and then places his left hand on the wire mesh, and uses his right to move the bridge of the bass back and forth under the strings as if playing a koto. The soundscape becomes airy, tonal, dissonant, and sprawling. It gathers into a chorus of natural and artificial voices that spread over spectra of pitch, tone, and timbre to give the impression of waves cresting on the surface of a sea of sound.

Aaron lets his senses sink into image and sound. He thinks of the valley beyond North Park, and the way the ridges on either side lay on the earth's crust like a giant fossil from the Dreamtime. Several minutes on, he seems to hear another ridge rise and rumble across others like a strong wind riffling a field of grain.

The soundscape shifts. Aaron feels foreboding. Tears fill his eyes, and he suppresses the urge to run. Enforced stillness takes him to the edge of an abyss. Inchoate feelings resolve into rage, and then an ecstasy of grief. He remembers his parents when they were cold with each other, and his mother was filled with yearning for—for John, it seems. He realizes that he has lived with John's presence since his earliest years, but never recognized it for what it was. Aaron folds his arms as if to protect his heart from the knowledge that he misconstrued his mother's state. He failed to comprehend his life with her. He thought that she was unhappy with the family and the end of their old lives when in fact she was longing for John as he now longs for her.

Aaron closes his eyes and opens his heart to grief. As John reaches the end of this wave of sorrow, the soundscape resolves into simmering, dissonant regret. Aaron releases his understanding of his mother, taking in John's experience of her instead; he is shocked to feel his love and John's as one. Opening his eyes, he shakes off his shock as John begins to improvise.

The melody rises lyrically to reveal a part of his mother that Aaron never knew and that is, presumably, alive in John. Aaron has avoided her sexuality as assiduously as he could, but realizes now that it was always in him, as was his father's and—apparently—John's. Aaron must have taken it in as the negative image of his mother's yearning. Aaron relaxes into the melody, which is at first like a long-lost folk ballad; then like a heavy metal complaint about the charnel yard of enslavement, war, and plagues; and then like a denouement of history expressed in bluesy, jazzy riffs that increase in tempo and rise to a sustained ecstasy of release.

Aaron recalls his father's state around his mother: it was generally angry and resentful, or contemptuous and disconnected—never like this loss or bliss. Aaron realizes with a pang that he has taken after his father more than after his mother; he has never felt what John is playing for—or with—another. His mother knew passion. That may have been the reason she used to say that heavy pain and loss inspire restoration. Aaron has embodied renascence—but only indirectly, through her.

Sarah places her hand on John's shoulder. He concludes, and then Sarah adroitly removes and wipes the disks, and returns things to their places. Gina helps her grandfather to his feet and leads him toward the door. His face is wet with tears. Sarah takes his arm, and John stops. He turns to Aaron, smiles sweet consolation through his tears, and shocks Aaron with his words, "She says not to worry, everything will be fine. She thanks you for standing in for her, and for letting her see that Rafa looks like Dan, but sits like her, laughs like her, and shows the same keen ambivalence."

Aaron is stunned silent. He is not sure what to make of John. Perhaps his creative state has overexcited his imagination.

John continues, "She and I loved each other so easily that I took it for granted. I thought that any man and woman could create a fire so bright that it would dispel all shadow. I didn't know how rare it was until I left, and lost the exquisite joy we had. Without my mistake, you and Rafa and Gina would never have come to us, so I can't regret it, but I regret spoiling our happiness. She and Dan never—Laurel and I never—couldn't—" John's voice breaks. "I'm sorry."

Aaron feels an impulse to join John in heaping blame on his shoulders, but pulls himself together, stands to take John's hand, and says with sincerity that surprises him, "Thank you for sharing the part of her that lives on in you. I didn't know her heart until now. I hope you'll take me as a second son, and Rafa as a granddaughter, and that Gina and I can become like family, too."

"I welcome the kinship," Gina says, visibly moved.

Doug stands and says firmly, "That's enough for us geezers. We can all be family tomorrow."

Sarah, Doug, and John exit. The door closes softly behind them.

"Did he mean what he said about … what Mom said?" Aaron asks Gina.

"He believes that your mom's intangible body—her being—lives in his."

"What do you think?"

"I leave death to the dead. What happens next is none of my business."

Aaron smiles. "There's something in all of this. I never had a sister, but I'm guessing that this is what it feels like."

"I feel that, too, an affinity—an unformed bond. I suppose it started when Granddad told me about your mother, and I came to understand that she filled the empty place at his table."

"How did you end up here?"

"Granddad told me about this place when I was twelve. I already knew that I was different—he did too—and knew that I should come here. I didn't know I'd become a complex-same. And I didn't know any of this. The enactment was a revelation."

"Yes," Aaron says, and then asks Parvati wearily, "Is it all right if I stay?"

Standing, Parvati takes Gina's arm and replies, "As long as you like."

When the door closes behind them, he takes a sheepskin from the stack beside the cabinet and lays down on it to reflect on his life.

Aaron awakens in confusion. It takes him several minutes to recall where he is and how he got here. Sitting up, he stares blankly at the instrument. He doesn't know music, but can transform this antique to better express being and becoming, and—possibly—to reveal something of the legacy that is already forming in his body and being. Tonight, he will see if he can use it to discover the singular transitions that have patterned his body and being, rippled out through his interbeing to every body and being that he has encountered, and possibly continued on through their interbeing to others. This is the network that he can draw on as he forms his legacy.

Aaron examines the box drawer of the instrument and searches the cabinet for photon chips. Those can speed up the analog to digital transformer, which he guesses may be an old midi. He finds no other period electronics—no useful supplies of any kind—and can think of no source nearer than the fabro center. He decides to scavenge his devices; his days as a communicator are done.

Aaron takes off the coarse shirt and drawstring pants that he had taken from one of the shelves in the lodge, revealing a sheer layer of clothing, the second skin that he has worn for nearly four decades: the communicator's undergarment. He looks through it to the chest hair it mats down and feels a momentary nostalgia for the nanotechnology circuitry that is woven into it, circuitry that confers on him the near-magical abilities of exchanging data, information, and knowledge—even the wisdom of his body and being—with anyone over long distances. It was this skin that turned his trim frame into an antenna for emitting and detecting messages of all kinds—from whispers of intimacy to the thunder of cries for consolation.

He strokes this second skin fondly, marveling at its ability to transform a remarkable prototype like this instrument into one that will express more of the human experience with life in time. Inhaling deeply, Aaron pulls out the rawhide string and pendants that he has been wearing inside his garment since he left the Amanas. He turns them over and considers them one at a time.

First is a hard-shelled bamboo case holding an identity key to remote databases. It can read fingerprints, retinal images, voiceprints, and DNA sequences. For weeks now, he has been using it to read his buccal smears for any signs of injury; he has found none yet. He flips through the rough, hard credits device that holds his few liquid assets; the smooth wand that reads frequency waves and displacement fields on all scales; the discoid nuclear tracer that detects particle emissions and mass resonances; the capped pin that measures oxygen and carbon dioxide levels; and, finally, the cosmic reader that orients him to plasma and particle phenomena near Earth that signal shifts in the conformation of space and time.

He leaves those pendants on the string and takes off the cork-encased vocal transponder that enables him to reprogram devices with simple high-level commands. He has already augmented it with the code Björn uses to interface with period devices, and that Aaron has already debugged and enhanced. He takes it to the instrument and pulls out the cushion. Before sitting, he raises his arms and tips his head back in the yogic backbend he uses to sharpen his wits. He then breathes deeply for several minutes before sitting down to recall and contemplate John's use of the instrument. After some time, Aaron concludes that he cannot transform bodily dynamism into harmonies as John did, but he can use his knowledge of the body—especially his sense consciousnesses—to bypass the limitations imposed by his ignorance of music.

Aaron takes a standard audiovisual communicator from his left pectoral pocket, connects it to the transponder, and begins to reprogram the analogue interface. He stops short. This period instrument would have been used with a mixer, a panel that digital artists used to create channels and mixes. If he had one now, he could amplify or mute sounds by source, reveal signals in noise, and discover resonances between channels. The panel would impose order—but of a different kind than John's artistry or the artistry of performance guilders, whose perceptions filter out what they deem inauthentic.

If Aaron can find a mixer—or create a virtual one—he will be able to recall states characteristic of various decades, and to recreate, analyze, and remix them across time. He can use any resonances he finds to detect and define biohistorical dead ends, lingering maladaptations, and fundamental alterations in states that nourished human thriving—including those that presaged habitat restoration and restoration of the body of life as a whole.

Aaron is surprised to hear his voice appealing to God—in Hebrew and then in English and Spanish. He plays absent-mindedly with the drawer beneath the frame, then pulls it out all the way to put it on the side shelf and open the lid. There it is—an old mixing panel. What a find! He need not spend the night searching for a virtual solution. He can connect the communicator and transponder to his undergarment, and his undergarment to the panel, and quickly reprogram the interfaces. A year ago, this task would have taken him hours; with the skills he has learned since leaving the Amanas and the anticipation that is intensifying his focus, he is able to finish in minutes.

Placing his hands on the instrument, Aaron closes his eyes and turns his mind to a memory of a family cookout during his early days in Denver. Something is in his way. He coughs. At first it is too close to see, and then he recognizes it as grief. He turns his focus to his throat, where sorrow has coalesced as a throbbing lump. He grunts and groans to expel it, but feels no relief. He forces a shout; his rough treatment of his throat adds to the unease that signals intense feelings suppressed for decades.

Giving up on memory, Aaron instead begins with his present state, which he improves by attempting to entrain his care state. This filters through the panel to the speakers and the wall, which shows faint blotches of blue and green. These calm him, enhancing his care state. Even so, he hears noise that—even though his ear is untrained—he can recognize as a high-pitched dissonance. He tries to sing, but stops when his voice intensifies the noise into a screech. Aaron continues to play with his body and the instruments until he discovers that unvoiced motions of his larynx relieve the knot in his throat and release sorrow. At first, it overwhelms him; then tears streak his face, and finally a long-held feeling of constraint by death and self-confinement gives way and he realizes with a mix of joy and terror that he is ready to cry out to God. He is ready to practice *hetbodedut* again.

He tries to do this through the instrument. Bringing his focus to his heart, Aaron opens it to the tunnel of grief that he formed when his family first came to this place and learned that there would be no future if they did not change their lives drastically. His father had responded as he always did: he grew cold and clammed up. His mother expressed feelings that had been too much for Aaron and Eric, but she had—over the next months—collected those feelings and used them to embody the knowledge that all of the human bloodlines on earth had been devouring the web of life, that life as they knew it was about to end. She then turned fear and loathing into action for solutions.

Aaron wills himself to awaken the bitter rage and sour despair that he suppressed then and to release them through his throat. The stubborn lump of unexpressed anguish hardens, and he laughs ironically. He is a communicator, but has never opened his throat or spoken from his heart. Aaron runs his palms over the instrument's wire mesh and listens to them form soundprints. They stir a memory. He and his mother were in the comm tower speaking with Sarah, and Aaron became aware of a blank spot in his past bounded by a dawning realization of loss, acceptance of change, and incarnation of the new. He can still feel it. When he tries to visualize it, he sees a rock and realizes that he is tense and close to panic.

Inhaling deeply, Aaron opens his eyes and tries to account for his experience. He visualizes his loss and response and sees dry ice. It is small, but if released could expand to blend with the air in the room and disperse far out into the atmosphere beyond. He had held on to the loss to keep it from exploding, and his grip had become so tight that it squeezed the life out of a piece of his being and shut it down.

Aaron takes another deep breath. He knows that this tumor of being is not the only hell state he has contained and retained. He has known this for years, but has never truly felt it. Aaron looks with trepidation at his response to the enactment and realizes that he is afraid of John, the long-unseen father of Aaron's soul. John loved his mother carelessly and yet so deeply and passionately that they had sustained a half-broken union and given birth to a cure that catalyzed the ongoing cure of the body of life. Aaron would not want to suffer what John—or his mother—had, but he may not have to. He may be able to turn his secondary suffering from a time debt into a time credit. If he can do the same with his suffering in the Amanas, he may have enough fuel to create cure states and discover his legacy.

Sensing another absence in his awareness, Aaron turns his attention to it and tries to use the instrument to fill it. He finds nothing. He takes out the gel, pulls the disks from the black frame, and places them one-by-one on his body as Sarah had placed them on John's. Aaron adds channels to the soundscape. To find signals in the noise, he programs the transponder to combine channels randomly and to play each combination for five seconds.

Visualizing John at the instrument, Aaron puts his hands on the mesh and listens for many minutes to the sequence of soundscapes. Eventually, Aaron realizes that John's influence may have been modified by others, and visualizes John with various members of his mother's friendship group and family. When Aaron visualizes Dan in front, John behind, and Randall and his mother on either side, his hears resonances, dissonances, and coarse, rippling sounds—like fingernails brushing across wide wale corduroy.

"I have a dead mother, two dead fathers, and one father still living." As he names his parents, his heart aches. Aaron is tempted to close his body and being, and so return to the way he had been before leaving his comm tower—neither dead nor alive, but in between. The soundscape slowly loses its features and turns into a dull, low background roar. He eases and waits. He listens to God. He hears the still, small voice in his heart say, *Go into the wilderness and cry out to the all-father, do the hetbodedut that you have been avoiding since you met Rafa.* Aaron's gut and heart are aligning. His flesh is releasing grief that his being is ready to pour out. He knows that when he unburdens his body, he will pass through a part of the valley of the shadow of death and make his way into the tunnel of grief that ends in the light and life to come.

Aaron strips off his undergarment, inverts it, folds it into an envelope, and slides it into a drawer in the cabinet. Standing, he runs his palms up his thighs and feels the resistance of coarse and fine body hairs. He doubles over and marvels at the wonders of his body. He needs no second skin. What fabricated skin could do what real skin does? The false skin has limited his senses and sense consciousnesses, divided his body from the body of life.

He shivers. Dry sobs warm his throat. Retrieving the sheep-skin from the floor, Aaron trades it for a fourfold one from the pile by the cabinet and wraps the tacky wool around his flesh. Half dazed by a flood of raw emotion, he leaves the room lit and the instrument on, and makes his way downstairs. He is startled by a desperate man who turns out to be his own reflection in the glass of a windowed room. At the landing, he stumbles out of a side door and into the garden where he pulls up the sheepskin to cover his nakedness. Near one of the benches at the center of the garden, he trips and falls splayed-out on the flagstone path. He is stunned and cold. Tasting savory thyme, Aaron opens his eyes to a mound of greenery that runs under his eyes and cheek. It is too dark to see. He pulls the skin around his body and tries to cry out, but is too exhausted. He contents himself with a silent scream. Tears streak his cheek and pool on the thyme. Sobs push waves of grief from his body. His eyes close.

"Aaron? Aaron!"

Aaron opens his eyes to a tuft of tiny green leaves. His body is cold and cramped. He is lying on his side, wrapped in something warm. Parvati's face hovers near his, and the sight of her warms him. He smiles, then frowns. He feels hungover, groggy, confused.

"Are you all right?" her melodious voice asks.

Her palm touches his cheek. Her gentleness thrills him, and he closes his eyes to better feel her touch. His pleasure ends when he feels a sharp pinch. "Ow!" He pulls up the sheepskin. His feet protrude. He protests, "I didn't drink anything!"

Parvati disappears, and shortly reappears with a sweating metal cup filled with cold water. She has misunderstood.

He shakes his head, then changes his mind. With effort, he takes the cup and gulps metallic, earthy liquid that tastes of the hand pump and the rock below. He shivers and comes to. "How did you find me?"

"A schooler saw you and took you for a sleeping bear!"

He smiles wryly. "It felt like Dirk hit me with his tranq gun."

"What happened?" she asks with profound and tender concern.

He drinks in her heart from her radiant voice and kind eyes. "This life is strange to me. I'm at home, but not."

She smiles, stands, and extends her hand. "Come!"

Aaron gathers the sheepskin with his left hand and extends his right. She pulls him to his feet. He sways, looks about, and sits heavily on a bench. He stares at his imprint in the wide lines of woolly thyme of the flagstone walk. His eyes trace the heptagonal shape formed by the paths that converge at the sundial-topped fountain in the center of the garden. He watches a spider scuttle across a dewy web on a moldy runner bean frame. He opens his lips to the dewy dawn. He wants to taste that dawn, to watch the sun rise over the treetops, and to feel the shadow of the fountain's tip trace the sun's course over his body. "I want to stay."

Parvati sits beside him. She conjures a bouquet of laughter and presents it to him. "On this bench? With us? On the island?"

Aaron's heart blooms a response. "Yes ... yes ... yes."

He listens to her breathing and to scattered birdsong. He hears metal clink on metal and forms a mental picture of the hospitality guilders orchestrating breakfast in the dining room. He hears thuds and clangs from the directions of the fabro and agro centers and imbibes the rising energy of their industry. He delights in the first ray of glorious sunlight as it gilds the rustling treetops on the crest of the hill. He glories in the sounds of children signaling the day with their cries. "So much beauty."

"Yes! We don't often see delicate puffs of white cloud in a pale orange sky."

Aaron looks up. For years, he has looked up to find either foreboding or reassurance. He can't remember ever looking up to rejoice in life. He must have done that when he was small. He must have immersed his body in the body of life. His mother spoke of it constantly, but renounced it for the sake of others, and he has always done same. He asks pensively, "Is Leilani right in believing that Pea's enactment belonged to her and to her sister?"

"Don't let them distract you. Anyone else would have been happy to see their grandmother recognized for playing an essential role in our history."

"There must be something behind all that distress."

Parvati says hesitantly, "I can guess what it is. Her consort—Wind Carver—may belong to the hidden group that develops new practices. Those can go wrong in strange ways. Leilani seems fixated on a static vision of her past."

Aaron frowns. "What can we do?"

She continues, "You can attend to your legacy, which belongs to you and to every life entangled with yours—including theirs."

"Entangled?" Aaron asks.

"Each perception of you leaves an imprint. We call that entanglement."

"I call it networking."

Aaron steals a shy glance at Parvati. Her green eyes are glowing. Her silky red-highlighted black hair is thick and shiny. She is burgeoning vitality, a living cradle of bountiful continuation. He is in love with her already, an old fool whose virility is waning before he has expressed it. He looks down at the white chest hairs that mirror the sheepskin, the bony ribs that show between spare muscles, and the bare ankles below. He is nearing the end. "I should dress."

"If you like," she replies with a glance at his bare collarbones.

"You don't mind my nudity?"

"We see many bodies when we study fertility. Besides, I'm celibate, too, and shouldn't be affected."

"What a terrible, terrible waste," he says passionately.

She asks, surprised, "Are you regretting your celibacy?"

"I didn't live. I wouldn't want you to make the same mistake."

Parvati looks away.

He changes the subject. "Your fertile states are free of the weight of decline and death. You overflow with passion and promise mingled with vitality and serenity. It feels as if you're surrounded by an unborn third."

Parvati gasps. She feels it too. The air is thick with potential. Her body has chosen his, as his has chosen her. She says delicately, "Your care state is … a revelation."

"You must use cure states for restoration."

"No. We learn to entrain our fertile states with strategies developed by field biologists and ecologists—and not everyone sustains those. We don't develop new cures for anything."

Aaron's heart pounds. Her being is joining with his, he can feel it. She is letting the process set its own pace. He feels no hurry, no holding back.

As if aware of his thoughts, she says, "I overdid the enactments. I underestimated your openness. I'll be more careful, now. I don't want to fracture your energy body. We can't always mend such breaks."

"Tell me truly from your core—what do you want from me?"

Parvati folds her hands and laughs breathily. "Everything!"

"What do you mean?"

"We aim to create a way of living that effects restoration free of harm."

"That's impossible. Every action has countless consequences, some of which do good and others bad."

"I know. We all know that the road to hell is paved with good intentions. But we have no choice but to do what moderns failed to do. We have to find a way to see the harm we do as we do it so that we can adapt in real time. The body of life can't withstand any more of our neglect, or of our careless or willful destruction."

"Every era succeeds and fails."

"Every era counteracts the errors of the previous. At the outset of the modern era, plague pandemics left humans with independence, conscience and responsibility, and also with compulsive, competitive hoarding that undid shared conscience and responsibility. We need to own and evolve and share virtues."

Aaron laughs and says pragmatically, "I'm going to need a consort."

"Do you want to share your legacy?" Parvati asks with trepidation.

"Would you be willing to share it?"

"I think I do already! When I was writing the enactments I thought a lot about pre-modern and modern habits of force and power. Working free of that could become our greatest contribution to fertility."

"That sounds like a vision."

"It's a problem. Solving it could take everything we have—and more."

"Will it take my life?" he asks ironically.

"No one's ever done this."

"I knew the risks when I left the Amanas. I may have been poisoned, you know."

She nods. She knows as well as he does that his future may be cut short—that for him, syncing with them may already have cost him most of the time that remains. "But what happened last night?"

Aaron smiles. "I modified the composer and discovered that my memories of Mom resonated with ones of John, Dad, and Randall. They're all fathers to me. That opened my grief. I went out to practice *hetbodedut*—to go into the wilderness and cry out to God—but I tripped and fell, and went back to sleep."

Parvati smiles slyly. "Is that why you took off the secret undergarment?"

"You know about it?" he asks incredulously.

"No one keeps secrets here—except the crazy experimentalists in the fertility guild. But I wasn't sure how much to reveal when."

"Things are moving very quickly," he replies, stealing a glance at her face. "My days as a celibate and communicator are over. I'm ready to move on." After a long pause, he adds, "Fatherhood is more complicated than I knew. I'm sure it will enrich my body and being in time, but for now it's … thorny."

"As you may recall, I took sadhvi vows. In my parents' eyes, that means renouncing all forms of sexual expression."

"Ah!"

Parvati can feel his heart aching. She reaches out to place her palm on his breastbone and ease his pain. His penis stiffens. A jolt passes between them, and her face registers shock. She pulls her hand away. Aaron smiles at the contrast between the memory of the composer, which revealed so much and so little, and her touch, which revealed worlds. "Is that what the vows mean in your eyes?"

"Here, our ways include consort practice. My parents will accept that if I keep our vows—and marry in a traditional ceremony."

Aaron takes her hand and kisses it. "Then let this be the time zero of our third. This is the beginning of my life, not the end."

8

Metamorphs

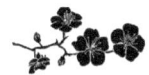

It is so dark that Aaron can't see the trail in front of the horse who is carrying him and Parvati north and east to the Kwakiutl Hot Springs pool. Aaron closes his eyes and forms a picture of the trail from the stillness between the branches overhead, the sound of hooves on the packed trail, and the murmur of rustling leaves overlaid by the quiet breathing of Parvati, who is sitting sidesaddle behind him. Aaron closes his eyes and enjoys the warmth of her palms on his chest and her thigh at his back. She feels more substantial than he expected as her flesh touches his.

He can recall holding other women, but doesn't want to. He has never felt love like this—the ache in the chest that stops breath, enthralls spirit, and carries soul away. He cannot take the measure of his feelings, or take charge of them, or accede to them. He can only ride them as he does the horse, with trust in the loving grace of the mysterious other in the foreground of God.

Parvati exclaims, "There it is!"

Aaron opens his eyes. The distant lights of the pool filter through the pendant cedar boughs that touch the ground ahead. As the horse approaches the lights, Aaron sees steam rising from the pool and disappearing up into the well of air formed by the encircling forest. When they reach the verge of ferns and grass, Aaron dismounts and leads the horse to an open place where she can graze. Gazing up at Parvati, Aaron finds himself dazzled by her beauty. Her sleek hair, radiant smile, and elegant, gold-edged sari evoke in him youthful awkwardness. He is almost afraid to touch her, but lets desire lead and summons his strength to lift her gracefully and gently down to the soft ground.

Allowing the horse to roam, he pauses to imprint this earthly heaven in his memory so that he can return to it whenever he pleases, and then takes her hand and leads her along the path to the irregular edge of the pool. She smooths the fringe of his riding leathers and asks playfully, "Are we playing cowboy and Indian?"

"If I use my arm as a lariat and lasso you," he teases, putting his arm around her waist. When they reach the pool, he hands her to a seat on a well-shaped, smooth log and summons his courage. She watches first in amusement, and then in surprise and alarm, as he removes his fringed leather jacket and wide chaps, followed by the shirt and trousers, and then, at last, moves to take off his briefs. "I'm used to nudity—but not yours!"

"Then you know how I feel looking at that kit you're wearing. You're dressed like a princess. It's a bit much for this cowboy!" He strips.

She covers her eyes.

"I want to propose this way so that you can see what I have to offer, my dearest love. I feel honor-bound to show you this bare skin and the life that remains in it. It is all that I have to share with you. I ask you to take me as I am to be your husband, consort, and partner in the legacy you wrote for me and the lifework it will inspire—trusting that you will choose what is best for you, and teach me how to care for you whatever you decide."

Parvati laughs behind her hand. "They don't teach this rite at the center."

"Take all the time you need to give an answer," he says, sitting at the edge of the pool and lowering his body into the steam.

"May I tell you in the pool?"

Aaron smiles and reaches for her solicitously. "Be careful! It's hot!"

Parvati removes her outer layer of clothing and slips into the water in a green breast cloth and skirt. Tendrils of long hair swirl in the water. She asks sweetly, "Give me your hand?"

Aaron lifts his hand tentatively. "My eyes are brave. They've seen sickness and death and they long for this life and your loveliness. But my hands are shy."

She very delicately takes his hand and slides her fingers between his. The pads and calluses of his hand join the contours of hers. The exchange of feeling through their palms is so intense that he wonders if her embrace will overwhelm him. Parvati quails, and he envelops her in a care state. She responds, adding a fertile state that cocoons their bodies and the space between them.

"I'm already yours," she says.

"Are you sure? I don't expect reincarnation, or an afterlife."

"That's how it is; we'll be one forever, but always differ."

He kisses her forehead.

She rests her head on his shoulder, saying, "I never understood eternity, but I know this is our immortal moment."

"Our first. Let's not close the door to infinity just yet."

Aaron sits on the sanded contours of a wooden seat. A light goes up. Oke Ten pulls a low stool up to Aaron's, takes his upper arm, and begins to inject red ink under the skin.

"What is it?"

"Seven lotuses. One for each lifetime of marriage."

"Red for blood?"

"Red for union at the root. Are you ready?"

"For the rite?"

"In the rite, you will leave ordinary time and walk with the ancestors and the descendants. Think of this, Aaron, when you lie with her."

A young warrior passes. He pierces Aaron with an unnerving gaze.

Aaron asks Oke Ten, "Is everything all right?"

Oke Ten looks up and, seeing the young man, smiles. "The young men are jealous of you. She was their teacher. You're an old man who's known her for weeks. They think you took advantage of your bloodline."

"I think they're right!" Aaron laughs. "I'm glad they're attached to her. They'll protect her when … I'm away."

Oke Ten looks at Aaron intently, resumes his work, and asks dubiously, "Do you know what to do with a woman?"

"Give her a man?" Aaron laughs nervously.

Oke Ten grunts disapproval.

"What would you advise?"

Oke Ten stops his task and looks at Aaron. "The way ahead is difficult. There are right ways and wrong ways and no way back. With courage and care, you'll find right ways—so you may as well enjoy her!" Oke Ten finishes with a laugh. Aaron is too distracted to get the joke. Oke Ten examines his handiwork and says, "Okay, one lotus down and six to go."

Fifty yards deeper in the forest, concealed by a nurse log topped with a dense growth of seedlings, is a small chapel where four warrior women are preparing Parvati for the rite. The tattoo, fragrant oil, and bark wrapping fulfill the traditions of the center; the rite itself will fulfill Hindu traditions. When they finish, Parvati looks at her image in a mirror. Her body is illuminated by bioluminescent and infrared panels. Her skin appears golden and her wrap red. She examines the symbols around the mirror that represent the island's habitats. In this rite, she will move more deeply into the body of life; she will join it materially and maternally.

A tiny woman with kinky hair cut in the shape of a skullcap holds up an orange sari bejeweled with mica, mother-of-pearl, and quartz. Her eyes move watchfully from the glittering baubles on the sari to Parvati's shoulders as she asks, "Do you want me to add this as a veil, or as a train?"

Parvati sighs in perplexity. "My heart is a covey of shy birds! They're frightened of me pretending that a sadhvi can become a wife! Let's cover them by covering me!"

A willowy woman with a narrow face says confidently, "His third will belong to us through you. Creating it is the work of a sadhvi—and wife!" She takes off her warrior garb, lets down her hair, and stands naked behind Parvati before putting on a purple cotton breast cloth and sarong. "You will keep your new vows as well as you have kept your vows as a teacher."

Tears gather in Parvati's eyes. She reaches back and clasps the woman's hand.

A broad-shouldered, muscular woman stands behind Parvati and takes off her warrior wear to reveal a snug yellow dress with a long side-slit that opens on a panel of red lace. The woman says, "And we'll help you celebrate them!"

"Aaron likes simplicity."

"What do you like, sister-friend?" asks a woman who

resembles Parvati in features and build, and who removes her warrior uniform to put on a kimono painted with colorful protea.

"I don't know!" A tear streaks her left cheek. "I'm not what I was and not what I will be."

"You don't have to go through with it," the tiny warrior declares.

"He's too old for you!" says the willowy warrior.

"He's a stranger who doesn't even know our ways!" says the broad warrior.

"Don't do it for us," says the sister-friend, "Sarah could be wrong about the legacy, or Aaron may fail in his lifework!"

Parvati laughs tenderly. "My past and future are his already."

The tiny woman narrows her eyes. "And?"

"He's kind," says the sister-friend.

"He's fit as a warrior," says the willowy woman.

"He's good looking," says the broad woman, "and he adores you."

"I love him and want to join with him, but … can you keep a secret?"

"Of course," says the sister-friend.

"For the allowed six months," says the tiny woman.

"If we can hold it in good conscience," says the willowy woman.

"If it's best for your being and our shared being," says the broad woman.

Parvati reveals that Aaron may have been poisoned and may have a short time to live. It is the first time she has spoken of it. The release of knowledge withheld opens the unknown future. She is afraid. The sister-friend sits heavily on a bench as she struggles to sustain her transformation of Parvati's fear and sorrow.

All breathe deeply as they practice giving and taking and restore their shared equanimity.

Parvati explains that she cannot support him in her present state. Their states have already weakened time and again during the enactments and their sharing of the legacy and lifework that she may be obliged to continue alone. She and he have even been overwhelmed by the intensity of mature love. She is not confident that they will be strong enough to form their third in the time that remains to him.

The warriors lift their skirts and kneel in ritual pose. The tiny woman says, "Tell us how to protect your consortship and legacy."

Parvati's face strains and slides into a mask of consternation. "I don't know!"

"I have an experienced consort and strong practice," says the broad warrior. "If you tell us when you need us, she and I will support you."

"I have worked with the poisoned. I can support his transitions," says the willowy warrior.

"Sarah is weak. I can support her dialogues with Aaron," says the tiny woman.

"I will persuade Oke Ten to give us time away from guild work," says the sister-friend.

"Remember," the broad warrior says, "You won't be giving away your body; you'll be joining with Aaron's, and pooling your time credits."

"Yes! The legacy has transmitted myriads of positive remainders already."

"Remember," says the willowy warrior, "Your bonds with your students are deep and strong and we can all support you in your work."

Parvati sighs in relief and puts her hand to her heart. She turns and hugs the nearest warrior tightly. The rest gather in a group embrace. Parvati says joyfully, "Your help means the world to me."

"We can do this together," says the tiny warrior.

"We can give you our blessings," says the sister-friend.

Each murmurs separately, and then all join in saying, "May we give birth to the next incarnation of the bodies of our community, our species, our habitats and the body of life."

The tiny woman holds up the veil again, saying, "Wear this train to emphasize that you're passing over a threshold into the future."

"And wear a bright veil that invites desire!" says the willowy one.

The four women take the corners of the veil, fold it, and drape it over Parvati's crown as a veil and a train.

Parvati regards her image. "This is beautiful, but it may be too much for Aaron. He saw my sari as intimidating!"

"Shall we try greens, or flowers?" asks the broad woman.

"Yes—flowers."

The broad woman lifts and folds the sari. The tiny one takes a garland of bright purple dahlias from a hook on the back wall and places them in Parvati's hands. The dahlias bring out the shape of her orbits and cheeks. Delight illuminates her smile. "They're beautiful. I'm ready."

The warriors escort her up the cedar-strewn trail. When Parvati sees Aaron surrounded by his warrior escort she is caught between a desire to run toward him and an urge to run away. She looks down as the women and men meet at the door of the Forest Sanctuary, and her sister-friend hands Parvati to Aaron. The warriors step back and form a semi-circle. His warmth comforts her. She takes his arm in both hands and touches her tattoo to his. The door opens. The warriors take ritual poses. Parvati and Aaron enter in silence. When all have entered, the door closes behind them.

Sarah leans on Aaron's arm as they walk down the path to the sanctuary. She is thrilled to have him all to herself on the eve of his legacy retreat. She hadn't anticipated that he would enter into the life here so quickly, or connect so deeply with Parvati. Sarah should have seen that coming in Parvati's growing devotion to everything related to him and his family.

Sarah says, "I usually use the Sanctuary for rituals—rarely for sacred dialogues like this. It's a treat to do something refreshing."

"I feel that way about marrying. It's a new life. I'm blessed."

When they reach the door of the Forest Sanctuary, Sarah puts her fingers on a disk in the wall of glass beside the door; it swings open. They remove their shoes in the entry and walk barefoot across the soft new tatami mats onto the rough central panels that are covered in woven twigs and set with metal handles. Sarah lowers the simple but stunning light-catcher and geothermal diffuser that fill the space with radiant warmth day and night. Beneath their bare soles they feel the warmth of hot spring water.

"How are you faring on the eve of your retreat?"

Aaron exhales sharply. "I'm beginning to get a feel for the context."

Sarah steps off the central panels and points to one of their handles. Aaron lifts one to find a pair of cushions in the compartment below. He takes them out and places them facing each other below the source of light. After replacing the panel, he helps Sarah onto a cushion. He sits on the other, takes her hands in his, and smiles heartfelt courage.

She continues, "Tell me about the context."

He contemplates this question. After a time, he says, "I should say my relation to the context: the body of life, I suppose. You see, before I left the Amanas, I thought I was exploring life, but I was really only lost in the architecture and algorithms of over-elaborate tools. I thought I was grounded, but I didn't know when I was or where I was in life or time. I thought I was doing the right thing, but I was just meeting the expectations of others. I saw and thought and did as my tasks dictated. I didn't see the big picture—didn't want to risk it. Now I'm ready—I think."

She nods, closes her eyes, and falls into contemplation. After a time, she inhales and returns to her questions. "What did you—and Parvati—think of the enactments?"

"They reminded me of the value of uncertainty—of admitting that you don't know something big and essential; of looking out for it."

"Good." Sarah adds reluctantly, "I should tell you that I made an error when I framed our history. I set up the founders as sources of inspiration and guidance and ended up turning them into icons. I've instilled idolatry. That undermines our New World self-sufficiency and confidence. And now I don't know how to undo that without disillusioning and disheartening our community. I'm glad that we've added two new founders who can serve as examples to emulate—and exceed—and to set the precedent of reinterpreting our history."

"You mean Mom and John?"

"Yes. I want to tell stories of the strong women and men we've taken for granted—those who struggled and persevered, and those whose mistakes are now holding us back at a bad time."

"What mistakes?"

"Everyone who came here early held themselves to exceptionally high standards. We had no other choice. Now it's time to ease those so that we can all act from conscience without spreading stresses and strains that feed our shadow side. I pray that you and Parvati will keep us true to our original lights—focus us on our meaning and purpose as they are now and not as we thought they would be or should be."

Aaron ponders what she has said. "Why not step up with Doug?"

"Neither of us contributed seminal ideas or fundamental problems or solutions. We're sterile in that way. We haven't given the community new life."

"Can anyone else step up?"

"If they were going to step up, they would have done it. They would have found a way to realize Reggie's vision of our species—that we would become like a system of the body of life that nourishes and coordinates it."

Aaron exhales. "Why not induct Pea into your hall of fame?"

Sarah smiles. "We thought of that, but Pea's contribution was to see that we had problems—like everyone else on the planet. She didn't create solutions. Melissa—and John—created solutions."

They sit quietly for a few minutes. Aaron expects that they will sit for a while and then leave, but Sarah looks out the window and continues. "I want you to see that we live at a kind of frontier here—at the edge of the known world."

"Are you saying that we'll be looking into the unknown future?"

"The future, and the wild. We don't know it; we're restoring it on faith. We're putting it back the way it was as best we can. You saw that in Dirk's bear. We encounter incidents like that more and more often; predators intrude, trees fall and crush families, intruders introduce fears and hatreds that prevailed before the year zero. And we have disruption without dissent, which could fragment us." She laughs. "Last year a moose trapped our children in the schoolhouse for two days. That's why we keep a perimeter."

"That's the modern way."

"Precisely. We have no choice but to sustain our boundaries—for now, at least—but I want to dissolve our boundaries and stay strong at the core. I want to put tribalism and speciesism behind us. That's the way to create an Eden. We can't just push back the frontier, we have to dissolve it."

"Are you saying that you want me to create a new kind of strength?"

"Yes, if you can. But what I was saying was that I want you to go to the edge of the unknown, to venture into the wilderness, to illuminate the way ahead as your mom and John did—before we lose our way or run out of time."

Aaron frowns. "That sounds like mythology, or scripture. I can't see how to make it real. You talked earlier about creating a structure—or systems—to replace you. That's a practical task, a matter of devising a form of self-governance. Can I illuminate the unknown by acting as a lawgiver? As your Dracon, or Solon?"

"Or our Solomon. Yes, but I think you would have to comprehend our core processes—and see what we don't see in ourselves—to find a flaw and formulate a suitable correction. If it doesn't suit, we may fail before the age of life in time begins—and there is no community that can replace ours."

Aaron stands and embraces Sarah. "I have faith in what you've done here. The Amanas have reinvented themselves for centuries. You can do it, too."

Sarah shocks him by bursting into tears. He smiles. "And so the son fathers the mother." He squeezes her hands, and she smiles through her tears. He waits patiently for her to speak.

She says, "I want to leave you with one last image."

"Go on."

"We need to imagine and train doctors of life—doctors who treat all of its nested bodies as one. Our species has not yet owned the pervasive fundamental sin of modernity and premodernity: vitacide. Evolved life now hangs by a thread because of our inability to take responsibility for seeing that the lives of habitats are the very source of our breath. Medicine can see that and save us."

"So ... Rafa and Parvati and I are to make doctors fertile enough in their creation of care and cure to care and cure for all creation."

Sarah pauses and frowns. "Yes, and to doctor life as it exists in time now and into the future."

Aaron smiles. "Not all creation, I suppose. No need to doctor the solar system, or the universe."

Sarah laughs. "Not in the lifetime of the body of this community. Life on Earth is more than enough for us."

She stands. "The warriors will come soon to perform the legacy rite. Parvati will come at midnight to take you to the retreat cabin." She places her hands on his head and blesses him. "May you dive deeply into the one life that began eons ago, and help us to help it survive for eons into the future."

Parvati's warm fingers close around the cold flesh of Aaron's upper arm. He gives himself up to her as she leads him out of the sanctuary into the dark, damp night and up the treacherous trail to the retreat cabin at the crest of the hill. He is in a daze. His too-soft arches scrape the rough rocks and roots as his body syncs with the moving front of time that consumes all lives. The love left behind by those who have gone before illuminates the void ahead.

Aaron's vaporous exhalations disappear into the night air. He stumbles and twists his right ankle. Pain sharpens his alertness. Limping up the stony backbone of the hill, he pauses to look over his shoulder at the scattered lights that reveal the islands of the Salish Sea. He follows Parvati into the cabin and onto a long, low shelf bed covered with grass-filled futons, downy coverlets, and warm skins. He listens as metal hinges creak, a match strikes, and dry tinder crackles, releasing pungent smoke.

The fire catches and illuminates the rustic interior. Aaron sees that he is sitting on a wheeled drawer bed that he will be able to push into the wall in the morning. Then he will be able to put down the hinged panel at his back and use it as a table. On his right, in the center of the wall opposite the door, stands a hearth with a wood stove inset. Above it hang pots and pans on pegs, and above those are shelves of dishes; on either side are a floor to ceiling cistern, cupboards, and two straight-backed chairs. Against the wall opposite him sit a desk and chair, cushions for meditation, and a prayer bench. On his left are wide blank windows that he guesses will overlook the north end of Saltspring Island, other Gulf Islands, and Van Island.

Parvati asks in a low voice, "Did you release grief?"

Aaron sighs and ponders. His mind is blurry, slow. "Some," he says. After a long pause, he adds, "It hasn't coalesced and left me."

Parvati says, "You took on a lot of loss and mortification. You relived your mother's losses; endured the shaving of your head, the anointing of your skin with oily soil, and the wrap in ash-marked bark; and then the legacy rite."

"It isn't that," he says, his voice breaking. "I can imagine that my legacy might count for something at some time. I may—with you—be able to serve the One—like Mom. But … "

Parvati takes his hand. He feels comfort. She is waiting for him to continue. He frowns in confusion, laughs strangely, and declares, "I'm coming down with her brain fog right now!"

After a long pause, Parvati asks hesitantly, "Is it the tests?"

He nods. "I detected something before you came. I know now that the poisons broke some of my stem cell DNA and remain in my marrow. I'm guessing that I have six months, maybe a year or two, but I have to consult a doctor—someone at our clinic in the Amanas who will tell me what is known … and what isn't."

Aaron can feel Parvati struggling to sustain her fertile state; then he feels her lose it. He loses his own care state. Hearing her breath quicken, he lets her put her arm around him and pull his head to her shoulder. He rests against her, feeling her crying. When her sorrow eases, she says tenderly, "We will live, love, and tend our third together. And I will continue—with your spirit—when you go."

He breaks down. He sobs as never before—but after several minutes, his sorrow eases, and his heart lifts. "It isn't fair to you!"

"We all look for meaning and purpose in life. Yours and mine are one now. The only life I have now is with you."

"You can have another one after me," he says. "With me—like John."

"It's too soon to think of that."

Aaron sits up and kisses her tenderly. "Let me know when it's time?"

Parvati nods her head. "Did Sarah tell you what comes next?"

"No."

"You'll stay here tonight, alone. Then I will join you here for three days. After that, we'll be free to go to the monastery for as long as it takes us to define our legacy."

A week later, when Aaron and Parvati have been immersed in love and begun to recover from grief, Aaron connects the composer to a black comm box, then connects both to the enhanced undergarment, and finally connects that to the skull-cap of golden wires that John is wearing. Backing away, he sits on a cushion beside Parvati. He turns to delight in the golden glow of her skin, and she smiles and enjoys his craggy brow, lined cheeks, and sinewy flesh. She delights in his gentle sensitivity and sweet solicitude, and he in her bright joy. Their feelings are intensified by their love of Doug, Sarah, Rafa, Yuko-Hyun, and Gina, who wait with them in keen anticipation.

John takes the virtual horn in his lips, closes his eyes, and places his palms on the mesh. The comm box hums to life, connecting John to the global network of contemplative doctors who share new, high-level knowledge. If all goes as planned, researchers in the Nile Basin will be able to use their data to refine methods of palmar diagnosis. Then the care team that is coming from the Amanas will join the network on a trial basis.

Sarah whispers, "Why the skullcap?"

Aaron replies, "When John focuses on a memory, the skullcap

will capture the activity of his occipital cortex and related areas. We may see what he saw."

The air between the composer and luminous wall shimmers. An image appears, initially nothing more than glittering pixels. Colors appear and coalesce. They brighten, intensify, and form shapes. Gina gasps. They are looking at a three-dimensional memory of trees, shrubs, and grass, and hearing a soundscape that fills them with yearning anticipation. Gradually, they grasp that John is walking along a macadam path beside a stream.

Rafa says, "I know that place! That was Cook Park in Denver. It's a skatepark now—cement and sand."

The view pans right and left, then returns to the path. Aaron feels dizzy as the image zooms in on his mother's eyes, which are clear and bright with delight. The soundscape fills them with exuberant joy. The image moves dizzyingly from her eyes to her mouth and neck, then zooms out. She is standing in front of them on the path with arms spread wide. The focus vacillates disconcertingly between her teeth and the landscape, then finally darkens.

"He must have closed his eyes and embraced her," Parvati whispers.

Sarah laughs, and whispers to Doug, "I remember him feeling like this when she walked into a room."

Doug replies, "Even I could feel that."

"She was beautiful!" Rafa exclaims in amazement. "Why didn't you say?"

Aaron says, "He's enhanced her somehow."

"That's how he saw her, and that's how she looked when they were together," Doug says.

The view brightens and lengthens, and the park comes back

into view. Standing, Rafa lopes past the composer and into the image. She stops beside the macadam path. The view lifts, and they find themselves looking up at glorious fall foliage dancing in the breeze. Rafa leans to one side, then returns to her seat.

Melissa's lips begin to move.

"No audio!" Doug protests.

"That's beyond me," Aaron replies. "She's ... telling him about my bar mitzvah!" he realizes.

"What's she saying?" Rafa asks urgently.

"She's telling him about my haftarah. She's bragging about my interpretation! She didn't praise us much. Instead, she worried. I figured out how to put her at ease and to help her relax, but Eric never did."

Melissa pauses. In the silence, Aaron sees that she would like to kiss John, but she steps back resolutely and takes his arm instead. John's view switches to the path and recedes into the fog of the luminous wall. After a silent minute during which Aaron and Parvati barely breathe, the soundscape shifts and a line appears on the wall. It resolves into a horizon. John's view focuses on a grassy lawn and jumps up to rest on Melissa's profile, her head resting against a rammed earth wall. She is decades older and looks pensive. The soundscape is complex. Aaron detects yearning, regret, and effervescent joy.

"Read those lips, bud," Doug jokes, breaking the spell cast by John's feelings.

"Where are they?" Sarah asks.

"Outside our clinic in the Amanas," Aaron replies.

"I didn't know he visited her there!" Sarah exclaims.

"I didn't either," says Gina.

"She's talking about Eric and me ... " Aaron's voice breaks.

Parvati squeezes his hand, and he steadies himself. "She doesn't know what she'd have done without me, but she's sorry I never had the chance to love like she did."

"And now you do," says Gina.

Doug confesses, "Truth be told, I wanted that kind of love."

"It's hard to watch without envy!" Sarah declares wistfully.

"I hope you and Doug will accept your feelings before it's too late to express them," Parvati says sadly.

An uncomfortable silence follows. Aaron is relieved when the air in front of the composer begins to shimmer again, but grows tense as the soundscape and melody suspend them between transcendent bliss and creeping dread. An image appears and reveals thick homemade wallpaper, then a bed covered with a log cabin quilt, and the elderly Melissa lying under it. Her hands are folded on her belly, and John's hands rest on hers. Her expression is pleading. Aaron states the obvious. "She's on her deathbed."

"She's saying promise me," Doug says.

"She's talking about me!" Rafa says.

"She says she's been praying for you every day since you were born, and her friends in the Amanas pray for you on Sundays," Sarah says.

Melissa's expression becomes desperate. She is looking into their eyes, crying. Parvati feels the group mirror her sorrow. The soundscape fills them with loving comfort.

"She's asking John to take her spirit body into his!" Aaron exclaims. "And to take her to Denver to meet Rafa."

They can all read her next words, "I love you. I love you. I love you all."

The luminous wall goes dark. The music stops. The room is dark and quiet for a time. Soon, a light appears in the center of the luminous wall. Aaron sees his mother's eyes—rather, the light behind her eyes—and her face—rather, the outlines of her forehead, nose, cheekbones, and chin.

"What's going on?" asks Sarah.

"I don't know," says Aaron. "I don't think it's a memory." He stands and walks to John, his eyes on the image. He hears Rafa ask Yukie, "Is it her? Or is he imagining her?"

Yukie replies, "Does it matter?"

As the disconnect wrought by this startling wonder subsides, Sarah falls back into her earth mother persona, Doug into his chimera of coyote and old goat, and John into the more and less that he is fast becoming. Rafa and Aaron say quietly, in pensive unison, "I don't know."

Aaron asks, "How did you make your breakthrough?" He is stunned when the mask moves and her voice whispers, "Urgent necessity."

"An emergency?"

"Need that gives rise to a focused, loving purpose."

They stare, dumbfounded. John disconnects his body from the machine. The luminous wall clears and brightens.

"You did it for love of her—and she for love of you?" Aaron asks John.

"And for our profession, and the millions of patients who suffered as she did."

"Do you have any advice for my legacy project?"

John laughs, then sighs like a bassoon in glissando. "Yes. Live—and love!"

"Rafaela? Can you stay with me a while?" Aaron asks when the wonder has subsided, the pleasantries and hugs are done, and the others are leaving with expressions of curious openness to the ineffable source of what enters the body of life through them.

Rafaela answers him by taking an ottoman and coming to sit beside him at the composer, her face patient and open as she waits for him to speak—yet she feels tense. Perhaps she is still feeling the effects of her rite, as he is feeling his.

"How was your initiation?"

"Life-altering," she answers succinctly.

Aaron smiles and shakes his head. "And what did you learn about fabro-trading from that?"

"There are real trials in life that have nothing to do with human malice. Which makes it a mystery and a joy."

Aaron lifts his head. They press palms in congratulations.

"Yours?" she asks.

"Difficult. I got to see my sweet young wife every day, but I had to come to terms with the weight of creating a legacy—which will help me to step up." He clears his throat and begins to tune the composer as he did the night he ended up in the garden. "And now there's something I want to show you."

"Oh!" she exclaims in surprise.

He adjusts the harmonics, attaches the discs to his body, and soon shows her his vision of his mother with her three consorts. "I think that you have three grandfathers through your dad, some more equal than others when you take the degree of union into account."

"Would it show the same for me?"

"Let's find out."

After they spend half an hour setting her up and trying a series of settings, a faint image comes into view. With delicate adjustments, they clarify a huge image of Rafa's mother with a faint, distant one of her father—and nothing behind him. She sighs sadly, then asks, "How about both of us?"

Aaron places his hand on her back, and they both focus on parents. The image does not resolve. He places the left leads on the left half of his body and his right hand on the wire web; she mirrors his arrangement. As he tries new settings, he says, "Try focusing on your dad and Grandma and you—and Parvati and Belatanu."

The image gradually resolves as Aaron continues to tinker with the composer; he also adjusts the focus of his thoughts and enters into a dreamlike state that he recognizes as open to his subconscious. Rafa mirrors it. Allowing a part of his focus to rest on the image, he is able to see Rafa and himself in front, Parvati between and behind them, and Melissa and John standing behind and between Parvati and Aaron. Dan, Eric, and Belatanu are missing.

"What do you see?"

She tells him: It is the same. She says shyly, "Belatanu and I haven't joined yet. He didn't think I was ready."

"Dad and Randall—and Eric. Gone."

"Yes."

"How strange it is."

"No. It isn't about them now. It's about us, for now."

Aaron removes the leads, resets the composer, and lets it go to sleep. "There's something else."

"I know."

He looks confused. "Sarah told you?"

"No. I've seen you checking yourself, and I saw it in Parvati's face." Her lips press together, and her eyes tear.

"Oh, that!" he exclaims in surprise. "Yes. I'm sorry."

She laughs through her tears. "Don't apologize!"

He reaches out and hugs her. Rafa cries into his shoulder, sobbing until she is all cried out and he, too, has shed tears. As she wipes his cheek, she says, "I haven't been able to be happy with Belatanu the way I should be. Whenever I get happy, I feel guilty!"

"Oh no! No!" he declares, taking her hands and waiting until she meets his gaze. "Enjoy him for me, not in spite of me. I have no regrets. I have you and Parvati, and this wonderful God-wrestling place where light and dark and life and death meet!"

She looks at him warily, sees the loving light in his eyes, and feels free to exhale, smile, and nod. After a long pause, Rafa frowns and says, "What was that something else that you wanted to tell me?"

Aaron nods gravely and draws a raggedy sigh. The emotion of the day has been too much for him. He will have to draw on Parvati, and she on her supporters. "Sarah told me that she thinks that what's missing may be doctors of life."

Rafa's eyebrows arch upward. "Isn't that what Grandma was?"

"I think that Sarah sees difference between caring for humans in and with their living context and taking care of the body of life with humans as only one element of it."

"I don't see how they can be different if life is One."

"Our species sees itself as the center of the body of life, as we used to see the Earth at the center of the universe. We aren't at the center."

"Of course not. But we want to care for people, too. Right?"

"Yes, but how? Look—here's an example. What forests need from us now is to eat deer as we used to do so that they don't multiply to the point of eating up the new shoots that are essential to the continuation of the forests. And without the forest, our species will die for lack of oxygen and other fluids produced or purified by the body of life."

Rafa sighs. "I almost get it. I've been thinking about it, selling clinics like Grandma's. But what does it have to do with me?"

Aaron sighs heavily and says tensely, "I'm not going to be able to change that in my legacy project."

"Okay."

"We're not there yet. We're not habitat integrated—as Andy intended to be. When we're integrated, we'll play our part in it and know how to care for it. Right now, I can only take a first step in that direction."

"That makes sense."

"I'd like you to write down everything that's happening now so that you'll have a record of it, and be able to think about it when you accept your legacy."

"My legacy! That's decades away—if I survive. What about Gina, or one of John's other kids or grandkids?"

"You are most like your grandma. John was the intellectual one; she was the grounded activist."

"We can't do this!" Rafa declares, jumping to her feet and extending her arms. "Belatanu's right. It's too much."

Aaron nods and shrugs. "I'm going to try. You'll be here to see how it comes out; I won't. All I'm asking you to do is to keep a journal to remember it by. Hopefully it will be obsolete when your time comes. If not... "

"A journal? Every day?"

"Quick notes. Things you want to remember. Nothing fancy."

Rafa sits down again. "You want me to remember you and our time together."

He nods, and takes time to let his tumult of emotions settle. "Like we remembered Mom tonight."

She hugs him tightly. "Of course I will. You mean a lot to me. As you said!"

Aaron sniffs. "Thanks."

Rafa stands awkwardly. "Maybe I should go now."

He nods and attempts a smile. She kisses his forehead and darts out through the door, which closes softly behind her. Resting his elbows on the composer, Aaron holds his forehead in his hands with a sharp groan. The composer wakes up, and he stares at it absently. After a time, Aaron shakes himself and inhales sharply, waiting for clarity. He turns his mind to the countless processes that enmesh his interbeing in the body of humanity, a body that itself extends back in time to Abraham, Lucy, and ancestors whose histories were forgotten in times unknown. Over all that time, humans made gardens and deserts, bred and extinguished species, and so shaped the body of life. Only lately did their fascination with death, destruction, and darkness threaten it. Only in this time do they have the chance to care for and to cure the body of life before the light of humanity goes out for good, before all of the Gods of the past disappear and become nothing here on Earth.

Aaron struggles for breath. He puts his hand on the wire mesh and prays for light and inspiration. An image of Parvati rises before him like a Goddess, and one of Rafa as she is. He would do anything for them. He would spend his life to sustain theirs. He will live—and love—and do what he can before he goes.

9

Eden

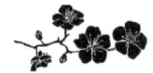

Doug leans on Rafa's arm as they make their way up the creaking wooden stairs leading from the deep-water dock to the upper landing of the Mount Athos Monastery of Origins and Endings. Rafa tips back her head and looks up at the forest, saying, "This is incredible! The forest at the fertility center is lush, but this … "

"This is an Eden garden. Part of this sector is ancient climax forest belonging to the old growth remnants of Cascadia. This part has been here since 1491."

"How did it survive the Great Drought?"

"Irrigation. The new monastics desalinated water from the Strait, built an irrigation system, and delivered enough water to rescue the bottom lands and restore some of the lower valleys—and to keep our oxygen-hungry hides alive and make it through the 2028 Quake and the 2030 Tidal Wave."

"Impressive. Inspiring."

The rest of their party—Sarah, Parvati, Yuko-Hyun, Belatanu, Aaron, and Björn—join Doug and Rafa, and Doug leads them into the forest. Birds sing them on their way; the air is fresh, tingling and moist; the lofty canopy draws exhilaration. Rafa inhales the fragrance of evergreens as they pass fir trunks fifteen feet in diameter, marvels at twin cedars twenty paces across, and watches jays rustle in a lush understory of salal, ferns, and mossy nurse logs. She feels that she is playing a pleasantly small and inconsequential role in this exuberant and exalted expression of life. Her love of the body of the forest intensifies.

The trail opens into a clearing. They see a campus of gardens, pastures, and buildings with hundreds of people working on the grounds, or streaming west into the forest on the old highway to the Pacific Ocean. Doug stops in amazement. "They really are swarming with forest pilgrims! No wonder Niko didn't make it to the enactments."

The others catch up with Doug and Rafa. Aaron asks, "Is that the cathedral?"

Doug looks at the massive rectangular building in front of them and says, "They call it the Abbey. It has a small chapel for members of the restoration orders, and a big one for pilgrims."

"Restoration orders? What are those?" Rafa asks.

"Niko—Reggie's nephew—and his mom Melanie co-founded them. They saw that the modern economy was working against life and started a holy order that renounced renunciation and took up restoration. Young people flocked in, put their backs into it, and built this pilgrimage center. More and more people are coming from everywhere to reconcile time debts through restoration as purification. Some stay and integrate into the forest habitat. That's why the Makah Forest goes all the way to Portland now."

"Are they restoring it all the way to Hadrian's Wall?" Aaron asks, tongue in cheek, skeptical at such ambition.

Doug ignores Aaron's doubt. "The Abbey is made of rammed earth with a covering of ochre and clay. This side—the north side— is the catacomb. Let's go around, get a better look."

Doug starts toward the east side of the Abbey. As he cuts across a goat-dotted pasture and between rows of mixed fruit trees to a reed-strewn path, Rafa asks, "Why use rammed earth, when wood is so abundant?"

"They vowed to respect the forest. See that stand of trees across the road, behind the aquaculture tank? That's the tree farm. It's mainly for bark, which is harvested in strips or sheets, so as not to kill the trees."

"Where'd they get the earth?"

Björn joins them, saying, "Right here. The soil was deficient for ag and the sodden clay would have shifted below them, so they dug it up, set deep piles, diverted the ground water, and pounded it into structures. They started producing ag and forest soil a decade ago, and then they put in the outdoor farming areas."

"Did he say catacomb?" Aaron asks Parvati.

"They have to put the dead somewhere," teases Sarah.

Yukie says, "They call it that because it looks like a catacomb. The real catacomb is below the sanctuary."

"It's more like a Japanese love hotel," Björn laughs.

"Or an old Pullman car," Sarah says. "It's an earthen bunkhouse inside the north wall."

Parvati adds, "Most pilgrims view it as a catacomb, and use it as a chance to contemplate mortality."

Aaron scans the road that leads west into the forest, on which crowds of pilgrims are leaving at intervals. Some walk alone, and others in groups of varying sizes. All wear gray wool shirts and sweaters, gray drawstring pants, and gray caps with earflaps. Aaron asks, "Is that—is that a donkey train?"

"Each pilgrim has the comfort of a bedroll and tent," Björn replies. "And each pilgrim train has a donkey train that brings food and returns a waste tank for compost."

"Pack it in, pack it out," Aaron says.

"They leave fish carcasses, and chanterelle mushrooms, some bird feathers, pine cones—things the guides consider as nourishing or expendable." Yukie says.

They reach the south corner of the Abbey. Doug stops and points to the south aspect of the building. "See how this glassed-in wall looks like the old flying buttresses? That's the hothouse—conservatory—frame. They grow all their own food. They even have a rice paddy and tropical fruit trees, and dine there in winter."

"Do they have a cistern?" Rafa asks.

"They collect rain water that runs into a central gutter, which feeds into the silo-shaped cisterns back by the catacombs. It meets their needs—including local fire control. See those towers?"

"The bell towers?" Aaron asks, looking at the four corner towers that rise above the roof.

"Those are drum towers. When it's dry for long stretches, they watch for fires and signal them with taiko drums. The rest of the time, a clarinet band comes out on the balcony above the rose windows at either end and signals the Pappas rule. It's a bit like the Benedictine rule. They're up in the morning at three for prayer or meditation, and do indoor work until breakfast. That's followed by leading a pilgrimage rite, and then they have plenty of time for restoration and purification work and teaching. The important thing for us is to listen for the clarinets that signal mealtimes."

"Why clarinets?" asks Rafa.

"You won't wonder that when you hear them," Björn says.

"Loud?"

Björn nods.

Parvati says, "Let's go in and find Niko."

They round a paved area with twig tables and chairs, and at the southeast corner cross a brick pavement with salal plantings in the form of three ancient labyrinths set in a giant triquetra of flagstones. Beyond, at the southwest corner, they gather by a ground map of Cascadia, with the Eden lands represented by dark earthen bricks and areas under active restoration by light ones. They stand there for a while, coming to terms with the patchwork of life and near-death. Rafa is not sure whether to be impressed by how many dark bricks there are, or how few. She does not want her cup to be half-empty. She knows that these communities have done more than anyone could have expected to bring the forest back. Finally, she smiles and teases, "This would be a great place for a skatepark."

Yukie says, "Yes! Most of us are sick of the labyrinths." She points to a high rock climbing wall on the far west edge of the campus. "And no one here knows how to set a decent route! And there's no bouldering at all."

"How does the wall work?"

"There are ropes at the top. We climb up and rappel down. The ropes on the back side spin turbines that charge batteries. There's one at every campsite to heat water for showers and cooking and pinlights. It's fun, but we could use a little variety."

"There's a project for you," Björn says. "Capture the energy of a skatepark."

"Skaters capture it?"

"A skater could use an arm to spin a turnstile—or land on a turbo floor."

"If an initiate wanted to do that, I could train her," Rafa says.

"Slow down, greyhound. This isn't a race," Björn admonishes skeptically.

"It's a race against time," Doug counters. "Niko needs more fabro guilders—and designers—and you could save time by training theirs instead of helping them yourself."

"Can't argue with that. Let's get Niko and talk fabro over lunch."

They continue to the massive west doors of the Abbey, which are glass and allow afternoon light to warm the thick cob floor inside. Doug leads them through a small side door into a vast, complex sculpted space. Aaron looks up at the soaring ceiling. After a time he says, "This is like—a Gaudi!"

"La Sagrada Familia—but it isn't a copy, it's an homage," Björn says.

"Don't they lose a lot of heat through the doors?"

"In winter, they lower bark tapestries to keep the heat in."

"Beautiful tapestries," Parvati adds.

They continue through the open sanctuary, past the altar and along rows of structural and utility pillars to a building within the building. It holds several stories of rooms: closed practice rooms, open instrumental lofts, an office with a library and comm center, and private areas for individual and group teaching and practice. Doug knocks at the office. A monk wearing the same gray garb as the pilgrims looks out of a round window in the door and nods. Shortly after, a man with hair the colors of salt and bark, freckles, and a closely trimmed beard emerges and goes straight to Aaron to grasp his hand, saying warmly, "It's good to see you all—especially you, Aaron! I haven't seen you since Mom and I came out for Reggie's visualization!"

"Good to see you too, Niko!" Aaron smiles broadly. "I

expected to find you in the long black robes of an Orthodox priest!"

"This is more practical—and supports our simplicity practice. And the fifty percent gray symbolizes our intention of abiding at the liminal boundary between light and dark—which we've discovered is different for everyone. We should probably have thirty percent gray for some, and seventy for others!"

"Do you usually have this many pilgrims?"

"No! This is the first Christophanic Jubilee year, and the Multifaith Council of the Seven Continents honored—and challenged—us with hosting a special pilgrimage for followers of the old time religions of the Mediterranean basin and surrounding region. Many choose to come while their land is released and shared out. That's why we'll put those of you who are not staying in conjugal rooms with the pilgrims in the catacomb."

"So you have pilgrims who are here to observe the Jubilee?"

"And to undertake reconciliation and purification. They started arriving in May for Ramadan, and more will come to observe Diwali, Hanukkah, and Christmas—and we expect even more for the various New Years and Easter and Passover. Some will be here for twelve months of purification, and many may stay much longer, until they reconcile their time debts through restoration."

"What is the purification?"

"We use your mom's methods—plus the practices of the fertility guild. I'd like to speak with you about it, but there isn't time. We've never done anything like this pilgrimage—it's been an intense purification practice for us! Fortunately, our guests take our failures as chances for repentance!"

"What failures?"

"It's been cold inside at times, and we've all fasted more than we intended."

Aaron says, "Let me introduce Rafa, my niece and Björn's and Doug's fabro-trader initiate."

Niko shakes Rafa's hand and says, "Are you and Belatanu ready to go up to your conjugal room?"

"What did we miss?" Aaron asks Rafa in surprise.

"Belatanu and I took our one-year consort vows just before sailing time."

Bel replies, "Yes!"

"*Mazel tov*," Aaron says with a big grin.

Parvati says, "Aaron and I would like to go up soon, too."

"Let's go now," Niko says, gesturing to a woman in the office. He leads Aaron and Parvati to the northeast corner tower, where they disappear up a wide spiral staircase, and the woman he summoned greets Rafa and Bel, saying, "I'm Crystal. Follow me."

Rafa and Bel follow the tiny, dark woman to the southeast tower and up the stairs. Rafa admires Crystal's shiny knee-length hair and her transparent and serene expression. Rafa would like to live as the monastics do—devoted to the whole of time and all that transpires in it. While the center is focused on life in time, the monastery focuses on the ontogeny and phylogeny of all creation. She hopes that will inspire her and Belatanu to create a third.

Rafa soon realizes that the tower is residential; on each landing, the square floor is lined by small rooms. Here and there, a door stands open and she glimpses through it a fold-down bunk, a writing table, and an altar for the occupant's personal path of discovery.

Crystal is explaining to Bel, "This tower houses the moss lineage of the biomonastery order founded by Niko's family—the

Makah order. The other towers are occupied by the bird, conifer, and arthropod lineages. Most initiates want to join the arthropod group, of course. Insects have never been so important!"

"What about all the other species?" Rafa asks.

"We belong to a network of temperate rain forest biomonasteries. Together we care for all branches of the tree of life in this habitat."

"So … the monasteries are for habitat restoration?"

"Those that follow the Pappas rule devote their physical work to restoration of the temperate rain forest. Those that follow the Kos rule devote that time to Hippocratic medicine—like your grandma—and those that follow the Pythagoras rule devote their time to theoretical work. All of us contemplate the origins and endings of many instances of creation."

"So … you're like the brain of the body of life?"

"You might see it that way, but we see ourselves as caretakers of forest consciousness, without which human consciousness would be too trivial to find the way to God."

"Isn't it trivial to care for moss and nothing else?"

"We care for the habitat as a whole. Each lineage measures the health of an area through the state of its phylum—or paraphyletic group or clade."

Bel adds, "You contemplate the smallest and largest infinities of time, but set your origin here, in this forest, at the moving front of time. You're more integrated into space and time than we are."

"And you're more grounded at the human scale. We ground ourselves in the tree of life, with the old Linnean taxonomy and Wuhan spindle diagrams. We've just begun reconciling our local trees with the work of the Mumbai ontogeny and Timorite phylogeny groups."

"You mentioned that last time I visited," Bel remarks. "Is it helping you to integrate your contemplative work and restoration practices?"

"It's too early to say. We have another venture that's more promising. We've joined the Aukland group that will be gathering habitat-specific trees and sharing restoration worldwide. Lack of seedlings of specific species is hampering restoration everywhere, and unlike the Finnmark, Aukland has enough microclimates to observe a wide range of habitats. If we can apply their findings on temperature insensitivity then our biggest problem will be that we have to impute species that no one ever measured, or measured too late."

When they reach the narrow top landing, where the stairs continue to the roof, Crystal, who is an unjoined celibate, gives Rafa a tight hug and opens the door. She returns to the stairs, places a palm on the wall, and turns to say shyly, "You can ignore the clarinet calls for meals. I'll bring your meals and set them outside the door. Blissings and blessings on your joining! As you say at the Center, love strong and live long!" She disappears down the stairs.

Rafa and Bel enter a large square room with windows opening in all four directions. She exclaims, "Look at that ceiling!"

Bel looks up. "It's really something in this light!"

They gaze for a time at the domed ceiling, which is covered by a mosaic image of the galaxy. The Milky Way, planets, and stars consist of pieces of colored glass that glint in the daylight. The borders and some parts of the planets are bright gold. They identify the asteroid belts and find the sun at the apex, within which is a trap door to the cupola on top where the taiko drums are waiting to sound the alarm.

"They said they wouldn't use these drums, but we'd better lock the door!" she says.

"The planets aren't to scale," Bel points out.

"Wouldn't be this beautiful if they were."

"Look at the tapestries!" On either side of the windows hang tapestries of many colors woven from the wool of sheep. They richly depict the habitat of the rain forest. "They're like paintings by Cezanne."

"Better," Rafa says. "And look at the views! And the telescopes!"

"And the bed," Bel adds contentedly.

In the center of the wooden floor, beneath the sun, sits a round bed made up in red, gold, and orange bedding with cushions of all kinds. He teases her by explaining the use of the pillows for various Daoist and Yogic positions, including ones that require groups. Soon, his pants bulge, and she runs to the window to look at Mount Olympus, the Cascade Ranges, Vancouver Island, and the San Juans.

He comes up behind her and presses his erect member against her back, between her buttocks. She turns, takes his face in her hands, and takes his lips and tongue in her mouth. He frowns. He does not know how to take pleasure in this. Releasing his mouth, Rafa moves to another telescope. This time, she turns and waits for him to kiss her. Her yoni swells. Her body is ready, and yet not ready. She could make herself ready, but the whole point of this joining is for each to learn to respond to the other.

She says. "Let's try conditioning our touch—massage, pressure, stroking, get to know each other's bodies, let go of our old conditioning, develop mutual interest and arousal and responses."

"Let's not get too technical," Bel says dubiously. "I need a little romance."

"Yes—especially here, in a church."

"You don't like prayerful joining?"

"I don't know what that means here. My mom's priest still considers sex a sin. Once you encounter that kind of fear and loathing, it sticks."

He says, "If we let our bodies get to know each other, and take our union one step at a time, we can find the sacred more easily. I hope. I'm not ... an adept yet."

Rafa waits patiently until he chooses to draw her close, and to wrap his arms around her back. She nestles her breasts under his chest muscles. They stand together and relax into each other until she breathes in as he breathes out. She says, "You're so warm! You're like my own private sun."

He kisses her. She allows his lips to discover hers, and then presses his lightly, and expands and contracts her mouth. He responds; he leads and she follows. It is like an old-time dance, like call and response. He finds his rhythm; she meets it. He kisses her neck; she brushes her lips over his. After a time, her mind grows quiet and her body discovers and conforms to his. He seems larger in her arms than he did before; his shoulders and legs feel dense as tree trunks. His lips embrace half her face. She realizes that he likes to get into a rhythm and to stay in it. He does not like surprises. He is steady, and even.

Some time later they hear the clarinet call, which is ear-piercing, and find a tray of food outside the door. They take it to the bed and eat together, then explore the four corner cabinets, one of which is a bath, another a toilet, a third a closet with supplies, and the fourth a fold-out altar. When they have cleaned up, he lifts her and spins her arched body playfully around the room, then they jump on the bed and recline on it together.

He raises himself on one elbow and explores her body with his free hand. Soon he sits up, takes off his shirt, and resumes his exploration. She runs her fingers down his breastbone. After a time, he says, "When I enter you, I'll enter all that you are and reveal all that I am. That's what makes it sacred, and profound. Physical joining is the end of something we've barely begun."

"We have the whole year for that, right?"

"Now that we're here, I realize how far we've come and yet how little we know each other's thoughts. I think I want to live here. I think I want to become a monastic."

"This year?"

"No, but I'll be thinking about it this year, trying to figure it out."

"You want to talk about God?"

"I don't usually use that language, but yes. I want to talk about what matters."

"Then let's talk about matter," she teases.

"You can't join without energy. That's the material point." He smiles slyly.

"Let's get to the heart of the matter, then. You start."

"I like what Aaron says about Kabbalah, about God meeting you where you are. That's what they say here, too. Do you see it that way?"

"I don't see God as a being; I see God as beyond being. I'm like a panentheist. I see God in everything, and everything in God."

"Then why did you close the altar room?"

"I don't see God in the altar; I see God in God-evolving creation. I see God in you and me and in the trees."

Bel nods and ponders. She feels his arousal as he says, "I

like that. I like the tangible—and the intangible things they talk about here, the fundamental patterns of non-generative forms of creation as well as generative ones."

"Yes. Old-time Catholics use celibacy to stifle fertility and to pursue sterility of all forms. These monks don't!"

Bel sighs deeply. He kisses her passionately and then, as their breath comes more quickly and deeply, says, "If you had no interest in the infinite, we couldn't touch it together."

"Why would you move here?" she asks, pulling back and slowing down.

"Their discovery of God is a lifelong and intergenerational task. They don't start with answers. They do what we mean to do—let the forest inform and restore them as they restore it."

"I love that, and I love feeling you like I did during initiation." She kisses him now, and he conforms to her.

After enjoying her for a time he asks, "Have you thought about our third?"

"I can't see our third yet. I can't wait to contemplate it in union after we've filled our bodies with the spirit of this place."

Sitting up, Rafa removes her top and lies down. He caresses her breasts with fingers and tongue. She explores his strong neck and chest and back with her hands and lips. She can feel their union intensify. As this accelerates, their energy bodies expand and fill the space between them.

She says, "I love the state you're in."

"What is it?" he asks as he straddles her and kisses her navel.

"Fertile! Grounded, creative, curious, solicitous—sharp and perfect for first intimacy."

"Are you ready?"

"No! I want your being to fill mine first!"

"And yours mine."

When their faces are transported by wonder, he asks, "May I?"

"Yes."

Very tenderly his little finger passes the threshold of her jade gate and penetrates it. He strokes his finger in and out and around the rim of her jade gate. Her fluids flow over his fingers. Their scent works on his senses. He breathes into his tension and relaxes into higher arousal. He opens her gate with exquisite delicacy and breathes into it; she relaxes into waves of higher arousal. Her labia distend. He straddles her and finds her jade gate with his jade stem.

"I'm ready—I'm more than ready!"

He lingers. She climaxes more intensely and focuses on the confluence between them, where the energy of their third will bloom. "I feel a third!" she gasps.

"Yes! It's time to join completely!"

10
Origin Rite

Shhh," Parvati says, raising herself on her elbow and pressing her fingers to Aaron's lips. "Here we have the luxury of knowing each other as we are and not as we think, or say, or do."

"As we are when we are one," he says ardently.

She puts her palm over his mouth playfully.

He wriggles away and stands, feet apart, looking down with burning eyes. "As we are, until we leave to see the hand dancers perform." He jumps down on the bed at her side and presses his palms to hers, saying, "Let's stay!"

"Let's go! They're taking the trouble to perform because of us—and their stories may inspire us, or change us—for tonight, or for all." Parvati stands and puts on her wool robes. "I need a break, anyway. My energy body isn't used to this! Its top is open—and empty!"

"I'm contented—and fulfilled. I don't want more—or less—of anything." Aaron slips on his pants. "But I'll enjoy seeing you in the role of sadhvi in a contemplative community, and remembering the best of the Amanas."

"I thought you didn't share their practices!"

"I was with them when they touched the infinite—and I touched it with them. I loved them loving God the way I love you loving Life."

Parvati takes him into her robe and embraces him passionately. "When the others go, we could begin our work with a silent retreat—for union."

"Mmmm. Yes! With and without joining. Your body and being keep changing. I want to explore them."

"Yours seem constant—but always new. I have yet to embody all of you."

"Exploring our bodies in motion will inspire us."

They touch foreheads, then pull away to finish dressing for the outdoor performance, which will extend late into the misty night. Aaron takes her arm, and they descend the spiral tower stairs as if unwinding the ascent to the union that can never be undone. At the ground floor, they exit into the cold damp air. She takes his hand and leans her head against his shoulder. Aaron knows that the rite will revisit Reggie's visualization of 40 years ago. He also knows that the monks believe in living each moment fully in real time to reconcile their time debts as they go, which would obviate the need to repeat rites, or to enter into dialogue with the past.

Aaron says, "I still don't see how they can be sure they owe life nothing."

Earlier, Parvati had answered glibly, "They consult their embodied experience, discern the time debt, and reconcile it. If the debt is old, they consult the archive." Now she wonders. She herself can sense when she is badly out of sync: she feels tension in her being that is like tectonic plates straining against each other until they release and shatter the calm. But she cannot be sure of distinguishing a single time debt from other ailments of body or being. "I don't know. Perhaps they perform this origin rite for pilgrims—to sync them with both our communities."

They continue west along the road to the forest theater trail, forming a single line with others who are finding their way by the mist-diffused pinlights.

Parvati clears her mind. She wants to be as receptive as possible to the rite. She has heard stories of the Origin rite for years, and Niko took pains to explain it over dinner, but she knows that it will challenge her, as well as Aaron and any other participants who are finishing their lifeworks and preparing for rebirth into the legacy years. The rite will plunge them into the full darkness of modernity, catalyzing the expansion of their beings and the extension of their metamorphoses. Those who are fixed will change; those who are changing will accelerate—if they recover. The rite sometimes shatters seekers. Like hermit crabs without a shell, they must spend their remaining time in the womb of the forest, or in some other haven in the interstices of the body of life. This is the reason that Parvati has asked her former students to support them tonight.

Fifty yards up the trail they enter the natural clearing formed by the storm of 2041, which blew down many forest giants. The monastics extended it to form the circular forest theater. They have a good view of it from the trail's end: They see a short, wide, central, glass-encased column of alcohol and oil fires that illuminates and warms the clearing; the monastics who kneel around the column facing the forest; the row of seekers that spirals out from the fifty-foot clearing around the center like an anchor rope coiled on a ship's deck; the cob gravel clearing that divides the audience from the stage; and the circumferential vertical stage that is both natural and built. Its inner lower face is a circular, shoulder-high wall of white fabric behind which rise the trunks of straight, soaring conifers. Behind them hangs a black curtain wall that muffles the sounds of footsteps and obscures the rigging, backstage apparatus, costumers, and others who enact the hidden aspects of the rite. Parvati thinks that she can glimpse the first group of monastic performers concealed above the curtain on a platform in the forest canopy.

An oblate—a member who lives outside the monastery— intercepts Parvati and Aaron. They wait and watch until all others are seated, and then take two reserved places on the outer spiral. They are facing west. The performer circles the participants and signals them to sustain silence, and to face east, the first cardinal direction of the performance. The light in the central column plays in the darkness, flickering and unpredictable. A faint, dissonant chord swells, reverberates, and fills the theater. It comes from the circle of monastics around the column, who are wordlessly chanting anticipation.

Abruptly, a circle of white-gloved arms rises above the white fabric wall. They swing back and forth like metronomes as they move counterclockwise around the theater. They are turning back time, one year with each swing of the arms and one century with each revolution around the theater. The chant begins as dissonant and arrhythmic and—as they return to a time before the destruction of the ancient forest—becomes harmonious but spare.

Abruptly, the clock and voices stop. The sound dies away. The arms disappear beyond the white wall. They have returned to a time before the known endings that came with modernity. At each of the cardinal directions, a cast of monastics descends from the canopy of the evergreen forest on ropes, and stops in midair. They begin to juggle fire. Moving as easily as old-time sailors over the sheets of a schooner, or as performers in a circus, they hang by one leg and arm and twirl lighted batons with their hands and around their shoulders, moving slowly downward at differing speeds so that the flames form the four phases of the moon. Their daring and skill are inspiring. On the surface, they seem content to express beauty and dynamic vitality, but Parvati knows them to be celebrating the vigor of the pristine forest that once thrived in this place.

As the performers disappear behind the white wall and extinguish their flames, the monastic guides signal the audience to all turn and face west to sit, and then to place the left hand on the right shoulder in front of them and the right hand on the leg of the person to their right. Those in front place the left hand on the leg of the person to their left. Parvati is pleased to touch Aaron's leg, and to feel his body as hers. A new chant rises: the origin chant. It is melodious and wondrous, and invokes daybreak, or a new beginning. It soon awakens the birds in the canopy, who join in and create a soundscape of awakening that spreads outward into the forest.

The chant dies away. Another cast descends in front of them. This one is clad in black and holding puppets, some large enough to conceal their holders and others not. The players at the center represent the Raven, a large shell, and tiny people emerging from the shell in the way of the beloved sculpture that they saw at the Museum of Origins and Endings in Vancouver. This representation is dynamic, though, and surrounded by forest beings drawn from the monastics' suborders. Parvati sees an eagle, spikemoss, a Dungeness crab, and several players that represent conifers as fractals. When the humans have found a place amongst the other beings, the players descend and disappear behind the lower wall that forms the circular stage.

The guides signal the audience to rise and turn until they

are all facing north, and to resume their seats. Beside them, the chant rises again and dies away, reminding Parvati that this rite does not follow the pattern of an inexperienced male in union, rising all at once or step-by-step to a single peak; this follows the pattern of a female or experienced male, swelling and ebbing again and again and reaching unanticipated bursts of ecstasy. It also invokes the continuing rebirth inspired by a still-potent origin story. Parvati concentrates. She wants to take note of all of the layers of meaning that she can in this viewing of the rite.

When the theater falls silent, its stillness is broken abruptly by the descent of another large monastic cast who form the backdrop for an origin tale from the polar region. This fills the north quadrant of the vertical theater with players in stuffed fabric costumes designed to resemble whitecaps and gusts of wind. These represent the spirits that reside in features of the land or in oceans of water or air. They display loving or hateful faces that signal their roles as sources of help or harm—that is, as holders of living time credits or debts that are liable for payment or collection. Parvati is glad that Niko explained the Inuit view as best he could, and that Björn likened it to the indigenous Australian worldview that joins temporality and eternity and a kind of dreamtime peopled by spirits and souls past and present.

"This looks like the body of life," whispers Aaron.

"Yes," she whispers in reply.

Another group of monastic players wearing fur and skin costumes descends in front of the ocean of spirits to portray the story of Sedna, a woman who attacks her parents and incites her father Anguta to take her out in his kayak and throw her into the sea. When she reaches up to grasp the edge of his kayak, he cuts off her fingers, and transforms her from a young woman into a frightening old woman representing the Goddess of the deep. Afterward, Anguta ferries the dead to her realm to sleep for a year before returning to the ocean of beings. The story is unforgiving and fearsome, a reminder of the uncertainty of life, which is greater in harsh habitats.

Parvati's heart aches to think that careless humans have stolen Aaron's future. She draws on the strength of her student helpers, and shares with him the augmented resources of her own body and being. By the time the performers descend, Parvati has recovered her fertile state and Aaron his care state.

As the origin chant rises and lifts their spirits, the monastic guides signal participants to stand and turn to the east. As the chant falls, performers descend in front of the tree trunks to the east of the circular theater. Again, Parvati is glad that Niko explained this story, which is intended to honor the origin stories of the east of the continent, as exemplified by that of the Iroquois Nation.

Niko's explanation allows her to deduce that the male player who appears to float on cloud wings is the Great Spirit, and that his gestures are conducting the chorus of synchronized movements of the beings that belong to an eastern hardwood forest, plants and animals depicted by synchronized aerobatic dancers dressed in painted bark cloths. Parvati notices that the players move as easily as her students do on the ropes and trees behind the school, using pendular momentum to swing across the scene, gravity to descend, and strength for hand over hand or shinnying ascents. A woman descends; Parvati infers that she is Skywoman. Her daughter descends next, and then the twin grandchildren who became the Creator and Destroyer deities, and who together begin and end all phenomena.

Unexpectedly, another character descends. At first, Parvati cannot make it out, and then she realizes that it is Shiva, the creator and destroyer God of her part of India. She looks in amazement at the monastic guide kneeling to one side, who smiles and winks. They added this deity in her honor, and her heart is pierced by this unexpected inclusion. Her pulse races as if she has been running. She has almost forgotten the ancient stories that she and Randall used to share as they sought to bring the gifts of the subcontinent to this place. She is so transported that she barely notices the origin chant rising, and the participants turning to face south.

Her heart opens to this next origin story from the Andes. The backdrop descends first. It includes beings from the south, the condor most prominent among them, each portrayed by a human in costume and supported by black-clad monastics who remind the observant that they are here, now, recapitulating and reliving a past that can be revisioned but not revised. The main characters of the story now descend contained in brightly colored papier mâché figures. Parvati's chest fills with love for Pachamama as the world mother is depicted in front of one giant treetrunk as a deity giving birth to the earth through the hoop of her skirt; she is also depicted in front of another forest giant as a wise woman who is representing the mother of all in a festival parade, and who is escorted by mounted gauchos.

Parvati fills with amazement as she and Aaron turn again to the west and resume their original places. The performers gather again behind the white wall and begin to move the clock forward in time. For a time corresponding to many decades, performers dressed in bark robes descend in a cascade of generations, miming youthful movements when they appear beneath the canopy and becoming dignified and then frail as they disappear behind the inner wall.

They hear the sound of a dirge chanted by a single monastic voice in the east. As time passes, the chant increases in volume as the monastics behind the white wall take it up. It is coming west. The sound is low, unnerving, descending, and seemingly inexorable; soon they are surrounded by it. It was composed by a monk who gave himself so completely to the community that he took the name Chantee and created no personal narrative of his life. The chant seems to Parvati to rise from his grave and intone through these monks, his descendants. The guides signal them to face east.

Parvati feels a chill. The white tide is coming, the cutting edge of modernity that will destroy every habitat and species— including habitat-integrated humans—in its way. A litany of watersheds in the Americas that have declined by half or more begins, named by watershed and beginning with the headwaters in Amazonia, which is farthest east.. With the naming of each, they hear a soundscape of axes chopping wood, trees falling, and wounded and dying humans and other species crying piteously or in rage. The theater is now dark in the east. As the litany continues, the darkness spreads, the chant increases in volume, and the body of life begins to die for the sake of consumptive destruction. Parvati has never heard so many river names, or felt so keenly the magnitude of the continents of this hemisphere, their steady loss of life, or the vanishing of the abundant resources of life and substrates sacrificed to its most oblivious predator: modern humans.

It seems to Parvati that darkness is engulfing them. Feeling a surge of fear, she notices that some of the monastics at the center are putting panels in place around the fire core, and so evoking the march of death across the new world. As losses and darkness grow westward, the dirge swells, and other participants begin to place their hands on the earth and to bow their heads, some pressing foreheads to the ground. Parvati also presses her palms on the cold ground. She is familiar with the quilt in the memorial building on Saltspring, but this is more vivid and immersive. Death seems to reach out to clutch them in its cold fingers.

With every loss, a death knell sounds. Parvati is not sure which is most difficult to endure: the inexorable loss of parts of the living world, the loss of light and hope, or the knell that penetrates the ground and the hearts of all who are here in this place. Together, they sweep away the mysteries that people imagined when they found the endings of Eridu, Ur, the Indus, Chaco Canyon, and all other dead civilizations. In the New World, this self-destruction was universal and documented in excruciating detail. It was efficient, fast, and almost complete.

Even before the litany has finished, another begins, this one of poisonings on, above, and below the ground, a list of water table desecrations, surface desertifications, and sterilization of modern arable and pasture. As the listing spreads westward to Oceania and Asia, Parvati stops listening. She cannot bear any more. She has gone as deeply into darkness as she can at this time without losing her way.

It is then that she realizes she has allowed her well of grief to divide her from Aaron. She steals a glance at him. He is sobbing, breaking down. She places her arm over his back, draws on the states of her students, recovers her fertile state, and shares it with him as she draws out his care and pulls him toward recovery. She is glad that she began to recover before the sliver of light in the west was extinguished, and the human clock turned forward to the time when all but a few parts of the remnant ancient forests succumbed. She guesses that he is overcome by the weight of his experience of the consequences of habitat destruction, and by the crushing details of rising temperatures and falling levels of moisture and oxygen that he followed for decades.

The chant ends. For a moment, Parvati feels an unexpected kinship with the late moderns who could not accept that they were doing harm, or that their children would be responsible for it. They were too close to their fears to conceive that cowardice and avarice were the cause, and were driving them to consume the future of existence.

Parvati gives in to the silent darkness. Her grief flows. After a time, it ebbs again, leaving her bereft but determined to restore their shared fertile care state. They are all cast up on the far shore of modernity, and have no choice but to take courage and summon the determination to restore and renew life now and indefinitely. The monastics have reached their year zero. The light reappears. Sitting up, Parvati looks at the silhouettes of the participants that it projects onto the white wall. She sees that every post-post-modern human in this place has survived but may not remain, like many cultures and peoples before them.

Now begins the origin story of the monastery, which is closely tied to that of the fertility center. It begins with the story of Niko and his mother Melanie who, with her polyandrous family of four husbands, initiated the grassroots restoration that rescued the bottomlands and spread outwards and may yet spread upwards toward the remnant ice.

The cast depicts Melanie's arrival at Sol Duc Hot Springs, near which she set up a canvas tent home on a riverbank and advertised a pilgrimage from Sol Duc to the high lakes. She drew pilgrims who went first went to Saltspring to study fertility and then to Sol Duc to purify their bodies by bathing in hot spring pools and then walking the Olympic peninsula. Some chose to stay and set up shelters and camps and to begin restoration.

The husbands came as complex-sames who lived together. All found part-time work in Port Angeles that supported the growth of the restoration community that was forming. All became close to Melanie and Niko and joked that they were her husbands and Niko's fathers. They took their roles for granted until the youngest man developed a strong desire for Melanie, and she for him. They tried to deny and suppress it, but finally confessed their feelings.

The oldest man, repelled by the thought of including a woman in their union, withdrew immediately to a hermitage at Moclips to practice celibacy and restoration. He remained a member of their changing family, returning once every few months to visit. The three who remained were attracted to Melanie in varying degrees, and she to them. They included her in their sexual lives. Melanie had no more children, but the community grew with the ongoing arrival of solitary or celibate hermits who integrated into the forest and restored it as it restored them.

When Niko reached the age of initiation, he became restless and went to stay at the fertility center with his aunt Reggie. He converted to Greek Orthodoxy and became a priest. Eager for ease and simplicity, he opted for celibacy, and returned to the Olympic forest to found the monastery. In time, all of his fathers came to help construct the building, and then they and Melanie came to live in it. They developed monastic rules, seeded sister monasteries, and, as moderns fled the struggling forest, expanded the pilgrimage and the network of restorers who were supporting the forest's revival.

The monastic performers enact this history in each of the four directions. They begin with the arrival of Niko and Melanie and continue with the arrival of the four husbands, whose interconnections they enact as a pendant dance. When they put on their monastic gray, joy returns to the theater and grows as the monastics recapitulate their restoration, and with the return of creatures and plants that had become rare and that soon increase in numbers. Light returns with the origin chant, and sanguine hope.

After, as they are walking back, Parvati sees that Aaron is troubled. She waits patiently. Finally, he says, "Four husbands. I see the way Björn looks at you. I'm sure you've noticed?"

"He and I ... I was celibate, and he put all of his energy into his work."

"You considered becoming his consort?"

"We never talked about it. We didn't want to take the risk."

"And then I came along."

"And then you came into our lives and changed everything."

"Do you want two husbands? Or more?"

"Not when I have you."

"You want another when I'm gone?"

"I haven't thought about it."

"It's up to you, of course, but I hope you'll consider adding him soon if you want another to care for you when I can no longer nurture our third."

When they return to the tower, she draws on her students, and invites their bodies and hers to ease his.

11

God-wrestling

In the pre-dawn darkness of the following Sunday morning, Aaron and Parvati arrive in the forest clearing of the Mount Athos Monastery of Origins and Endings. They are chilled by the damp air, warmed by the fire in their flesh, and open to the inspiration that permeates the breath of the forest yet seems to evade them shyly whenever they draw near. They enter the wall of white fabric panels that the monastics placed around the fire tower, light the fuel at the top level of the tower, and welcome the second week of their retreat with a chant that rouses them from sleepy disorientation and raises them to an ecstasy that brightens their view of the luminous morning mist.

As the sun runs low along the horizon behind the translucent ceiling of sky, Aaron and Parvati digest memories that linger in their depths; penetrate the living past in dialogue; join the full extent of their beings to the far reaches of their shared interbeing in union; and open to the future in contemplation. They invite the new to emerge from the unseen and unknown. As they have all week, they open and open again until they are as defenseless as lambs and ready to spend all the resources that remain to them on revelation and renaissance.

When the light above dims and darkness rises around them, they light the fires in the lower levels of the tower and circle it arm in arm beside their shadows. As the air grows crisper and drains their heat, Aaron feels his energy sink into the deep end of a dark pool of sacrificial blood. He would give life more. He would give it his last fertile imaginings. He would draw from his body all that the earth has given him and turn it into a legacy that will help to sustain life into the future. He would make good on the best of his ancestors and on those who are his kin—or who are akin to him now.

He feels the subtle processes that have carried him through time dispersing into a miasma that in turn disappears into nothing. Despair enters his flesh as a gas penetrates a liquid: steadily, speedily, smoothly. He is ready to let these ephemeral threads that have bound him to life attenuate like golden wires that have grown so slight as to break—but he waits. He will hold on to the light of his life for a little while longer.

Stopping his intangible downward spiral, Aaron pulls Parvati close until she is looking over his shoulder and he over hers. He whispers in her ear, "I think I know where to find what we're looking for. I think you're going to have to let me fall."

"Fall? What do you mean?"

"Into darkness and chaos. Into shadow. Into my shadow, the one that will become forever dark when my light goes out. It's mine to transform, and I can't see it when your love is holding me to life."

"I don't understand."

"I don't either. But I think it's time for me to die before I die, to leave *Pardes*, to fall from the grace of our innocent desire to give all. I never heard Reggie's words until now. Now is the time of my harrowing. Now is the time when I follow Mom into the depths."

Aaron leads Parvati to the other side of the flaming tower

and pulls the cot to the eastern point of their cylindrical space. He sits on it sideways and gently guides her on top of him. He lies down. She straddles him, sucks his tongue, and says tenderly, "Your body is wasting. We should care for it while we can."

"Tomorrow we will. Tomorrow, we'll take a feasting day and enjoy the cozy room in the tower. Tonight you'll let me fall, and I'll dream dark dreams, and you'll go to the lodge and contemplate and dialogue with Björn."

"No, I won't," she says firmly. "You have too much faith in your time debt."

He shakes his head and opens his mouth mutely. He is growing weak, he is desperate. She is not sure what to do. His illness is obscuring his being in her eyes.

She asks, "Would you leave me before we know our third?"

"No. No! That's why I have to descend, to harrow my being—"

Parvati manages a warm laugh. "Giving your life before you give our third life will not help. I will let you fall tonight, but not farther than is safe. And then we will go to the tower to feast and write and practice an equal ascent. We will—together—find light and life to offset the ravages of your ordeal."

He looks unconvinced. Before he can speak, she presses a finger across his lips for silence and laughs with more true delight as she says, "Our community is strong. Its next step may be close to what we now imagine to be *Pardes*—paradise. Trust in that." She touches his crown with her palms and draws energy up to hers. "Close your eyes. Do you see it?"

He obeys. "White crown light?"

"Yes. Remember, it is always there, and I can always help you find it."

He nods and embraces her tightly. "Thank you, mother of my third."

"Stay with me and father my third."

"I will."

"It is ours equally. Remember to decide with me, not for me."

"When the time is right."

"Yes. When it is right. Which may not be for months or years. We have only just begun."

He sighs deeply. "It seems maddeningly slow."

"As the art of life is. We cannot force it."

"We should not."

Finally, Aaron relaxes and falls quickly into a deep sleep. Parvati lies awake to draw and share energy and to bless him, pleased that the crisis is averted and pensive about the power of his passion to create and destroy in one.

The next Friday, when Aaron is rested and stronger, he persuades Parvati to support him in a night of God-wrestling on the Jewish Sabbath, called Shabbat, which begins at sundown. She can tell that the idea of doing so lifts his being and strengthens his body, and though she is concerned that he may push himself too far, she can see that he is confident that his spirit will be stronger on the Sabbath and that he is eager to enter what his family saw as its palace in time. He is primed, he believes, to touch the ephemeral as well as the eternal—and to avoid a precipitous or unstoppable descent.

After a good dinner, and a time of contemplation in the forest clearing that extends into the twilight, they go to their cot, and he lies down.

Parvati pulls a thick bark blanket from beneath the cot, kisses his navel, cocoons him in rough warmth, and, after one last long kiss on the mouth, says, "I will leave now, but I will not go far, and when I come back I will stay with you until your flesh is cold and your being rests in mine."

As she disappears toward the monastery, Aaron feels a stab of regret. He would rather be with her than be true to the world. Perhaps he has not come to grips with his legacy, because he is trying to delay what lies beyond it. He will have to let slip fear and every other thread of meaning that binds him. He cannot hold back. He can only let time turn his life inside out and shake out those obscure treasures pocketed in the recesses of his flesh.

He lets order go. His mind races along old tracks to nowhere. He forgets his purpose. That will not do. He must keep his purpose before him. He would father the continuation of a kindred that is bringing its corner of the world back to life. Holding the future before his mind's eye, Aaron invites his subconscious to open. After a time that is like floating in nothingness, he sees that he is afraid to be like his mother. He tried to ease her pain for years and eventually blocked it out. This, too, must open.

Aaron struggles, and after a time turns his mind's eye to the patch of past that holds his fear of pain. All that his father was unable to do is connected with that patch. He opens his hand as if to take his father's and enters it. After terror come sensations that he has not reconciled and that he can no longer afford to reconcile. These may die with his body, or he may leave them to Rafa, or to those concepto guilders and warriors and restorationists who reconcile vague and disowned errors of the past. Floating over these time debts, bypassing his embodiment of his parents' pain and their desire to bar him from their pain, he looks to other narrow places.

His focus moves on through his infinite network of cross-linked, accidentally indexed, fluid memories, noting some that seem fixed and fateful, others that appear nonsensical, and still other highly charged yet inchoate memories that he has yet to reconcile. He recalls his mother describing illness as a perpetual crucifixion and resurrection. She seems to have meant that light and life come from pain and loss. Her pain and loss flood his flesh.

Aaron sinks into nothingness. He falls asleep, leaving awareness as he will do at the end. Dreams come. He drifts in and out of them, aware enough somehow to register whole-body pain and to monitor surprise and horror. His memory leaps to his studies. His mind races along circuits, jumps gaps, and encounters the systems of thought that formed solid state physics. He follows them into the depths of atoms and into the singularities of black holes. He is aware that he is still curious about the patterns he perceives, and that his mind sustains patterns that give rise to material inventions just as Parvati's mind sustains patterns that give rise to narratives and meanings for life and continuation. Aaron is heartened by the realization that he was right: Björn is the one to follow as her consort. He, too, will be able to ground her narrative in material invention.

Sinking through the mesh of circuits and networks into the depths of matter and energy, he sees an image: an array of atoms around which electrons flow. He recognizes it as a metal crystal. He is a child of understanding and flesh; he embodies what he sees. He is the metal crystal, though his memory of it is spread throughout his nervous system. He could not have accessed the memory on purpose; it is too dispersed, too deep, too pervasive. It permeates flesh and is permeable to awareness. He would watch its beauty, but he feels it more than he sees it. He feels a stab of regret. As Rilke said, the time of the eyes is ended, and yet he will mourn every true miracle witnessed through the telescopes and microscopes of modernity. The pain of loss deepens.

Aaron continues sinking into embodied memory and recognizes that this experience of metal may die with him. His flesh can recreate this time asset, but when that flesh decomposes, his assets will be untethered and held by others—or by none. No one will be able to recreate them; they are made of his life experience. If he is to be fertile, he must extract its pattern and its meaning. He must win the race with death. The path of failure deepens the pain that he has gathered and would use up.

He knows that he cannot impose the pattern of this image on whatever phenomenon he would. Like Cinderella's slipper, this human-made model must fit a living process so perfectly as to fit no other better. It must also move from his living body to Parvati's—or into the space between them. He is certain that the pattern he is seeing is the source—or perhaps one source—of his peculiar fertility, and that he must present it to his subconscious mind as a puzzle. He must allow the part of his understanding that matches patterns to fit this one to a living process, and thereby structure the embodied shared interbeing of the community.

He does not want to err in this task. Should his mind mismatch the pattern and the process, he will obscure their third and they may give birth to nothing. Used wrongly, the pattern might confuse and confound the community and speed its degradation or interrupt the lineage of the legacy that his mother carried as dissent, and that may go back to the Swedenborgians or to the Lollards or to the hunters of mastodons. He feels a sudden passion to allow it to work through him, but how?

Awakening, Aaron calms his mind and contemplates the metal crystal he has seen. After a time, he sees the nuclei in the crystal as the guilds of the communities. Rafa and the other initiates circulate around like electrons, moving from one guild to the next. His eyes shoot open. *I have it!* The guilds are dividing the community! It is fragmenting all too soon. There must be a guild of the whole that contains all guilds and all who do not belong to guilds, and it must make important decisions and mend division transparently through dissent and consensus. Guilds can become training programs that the young pass through on their way to something else, as Rafa plans to do. And initiates must be free to combine them so that there are as many guilds of one or more as are needed to allow people to act conscientiously for the good of the body of life. Pain and loss lift with success.

Aaron can barely contain his excitement. He has to tell Parvati so that she and Björn can hold the legacy when they are consorts. He has to tell Niko and the others who can pray for them to keep the strength and inspiration to engage all their time assets.

Bright crown light nearly blinds Aaron and blocks his residual suffering as he closes the vents of the fire tower, wraps himself in his bark blanket, and fumbles for his pinlight. He rushes out across the clearing, along the trail, and down the road that divides him from Parvati. When he bursts into their room in the tower, he is dismayed to find her crying into her pillow. He rushes to sit at her side and places his hand gently on her shoulder. She wipes her face and turns to him, eyes averted.

"I'm sorry!" Aaron says, kissing Parvati's forehead. "I should have known that you might fall, too."

She gazes into his eyes. Her tears flow freely as she says, "I don't mind falling for the sake of this ordeal, but I don't want to fall again too soon."

"You didn't tell me you were holding a source of darkness."

"I became a sadhvi to reconcile certain memories, but they were too deeply rooted, and now they've grown stronger, and they're wasting my heart the way your poison is wasting your flesh."

"They're weak, then. Your heart is as life-giving as this forest." Aaron kisses her forehead again and asks, "What's troubling it?"

She turns her cheek and rests it on his chest. "The branding suicides."

"How did they affect you?" he asks in surprise.

"They came right around the globe to India."

"Go on."

"The old economy was in its last years, and the media had gone into decline, and young people who relied on commercials to lift their spirits turned to local economies. Some gave young people faith in the future, but many caused despair—including the ones led by my grandfather, who manipulated the young with aggression and fear. That pushed them to lose faith in life."

Aaron hugs Parvati close and waits for her to continue.

"He held to old ideas of caste and religion, and looked down on societies where the young were giving up. He told his joint family that such a thing could never happen in India among Parsees or Hindus of high caste. So he built a shopping mall near our joint family house. It was one of the few places where the young could gather outside the home. He had stores that he filled with glittering brand clothing and accessories and showed films in which young women who bought them gained love and good fortune."

Parvati stops and sighs haltingly. Aaron says gently, "Go on."

"I haven't spoken of this for years now!"

"Take your time."

After a long pause, Parvati continues, "At first he used his children, too. He bought them all very expensive personal items to boost sales. When sales fell, he stopped giving them things. Their new friends began to taunt them. Grandfather explained that their new friends came from weak families, that ours was gaining in wealth and we would all get good educations, find work, and marry well."

Parvati sighs again and continues, "My father and aunts and uncles were miserable and angry and began to defy Grandfather. When he made their lives even more miserable, they began to sneak out at night. Two of my aunts began to exchange sex for brand goods, and then for drugs. When one was abducted and held for ransom, he paid, but then locked them in or out, depending on what they had done. Then ... then ... four of my aunts and cousins ... suicided."

Having managed to say the words, Parvati cries for several minutes, and then continues in an even tone, "My father's older brother tried to hold the family together, but gave up and sold the joint home. My father went to Zanzibar for a time, and then out to Fiji to work for a distant cousin. He made connections in Australia that he was able to build into a trading route. We lived on the boat, you see, and used very little fuel, so he was in a good position to sustain trade in spices, teas and fabrics."

"And then you came here."

"First he met my mother in Fiji. She was a natural tantrika, and helped my father sustain the heart of our culture on very little money. Traditionally, Indian parents work for material wealth until their legacy years, but mine lived on faith in life. They were renunciates even while they were trading. As I was growing up, I followed them in worrying less and less about material wealth and more and more about recognizing and weaving into our culture the yogic practices of other cultures around the globe—as Gandhi did. They did what you might call deep networking around the Pacific and Indian Oceans, and then brought us here to see the forest."

"Why did you stay? Was it for the forest? Or for the purification?"

"The forest and the pilgrimage eased our hearts, but I would have gone on with my parents if I hadn't met Randall. He was doing what we were doing, but had gone far deeper. I saw that if I took him as my root guru and became part of his large body, I could do more than I had hoped to do to shift the balance of destruction and creation toward restoration of the body of life."

"His large body?"

"You've spoken of the body of Christ in the Amanas; each of our great gurus has a large body—a community that keeps his teachings alive when the guru dies."

"I see why you wanted a traditional wedding. You're still Hindu."

"I used to try to follow the river of the old religion, but I have trouble finding its course. It's disappearing in reedy swamps, cutting new channels, meandering through oxbows. I can't read its currents or its course, or trust my elders to read it, and so I go where the spirit leads me—like Colette."

"I feel that I've left the old ways behind—which means bringing forward the best of the past."

"In this case, we're doing the same but languaging it

differently, I think. Hinduism and Judaism can evolve quite naturally, if we let them."

Aaron considers this for a while, and then says, "One thing I learned from my family is that we have to be very careful when we interfere with evolution—even the evolution of a personal narrative. We like to draw lines and create categories that make us feel secure but that also obscure reality. Better to have no tradition than use it to fool ourselves."

Parvati exhales deeply and then takes his face between her hands. She kisses him sweetly on the lips and says, "Which is why we should put all of this behind us now and focus on your legacy."

Aaron pauses and says thoughtfully, "Our legacy. Something in your old sorrow will tell us what work lies ahead of us, which is probably the work that lies ahead of the community."

"It seems too specific to me."

"Perhaps, let's let it rest for now and see what happens." He takes her hand and says, "I have good news! I think I was able to diagnose the body of the community, as Mom would have wanted."

Her mouth drops open, then Parvati says urgently, "Tell me!"

"The guilds are becoming more separate and set in their ways. That's compartmentalizing the kindred and causing fixity and stasis which in turn cause division and decline. That's the reason we are out of sync. That's why vision, discovery, and social evolution are stalling."

"You think the guilds are patterning problems instead of solving them?"

"I think the gaps around the guilds are where the problems are hidden."

"And the solutions?" Parvati asks.

He takes her other hand in his and touches foreheads. "In us and between us."

"All we have to do is give birth to our third."

"Yes, that's all." He laughs.

12

Discovery

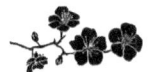

By the next Friday afternoon, they have talked through the obstacles of new guilds and old money and religions and force and tribalism and competition, and agree that old boundaries are fading and will continue to do so without more attention. They also agree that the new guild boundaries, in contrast, are directly in their way, and beg alteration or dissolution.

That evening, the sky is clear but for scudding mists, and they are able to discern two early stars and observe an earlier Sabbath with candles and *Kiddush* and kugel. After enjoying a lively dinner with Niko and other new friends, Aaron says, "Let's go up and use the composer. I can show you Mom, and my three fathers."

"Not four?" Niko laughs.

"Only three," Aaron replies, happy in the realization that Shabbat and new friends infuse him with enough new life to allow each moment to seem immortal.

Aaron enters the chamber, giving the bed a little pat as he passes, as if to draw inspiration from union with his beloved. He sits on the zabuton cushion in front of the mobile composer that they brought from the Center. Sarah had shown him all of the composers that community members had made, and Aaron disassembled them and created a new one for his purposes. The table it rests on, with the wire-wrapped rosewood frame, faces a luminous screen that they brought and placed in front of a tapestry panel.

Parvati comes to sit behind him, pressing her left palm into the secret chakra below his navel and placing her right palm on the back of her left hand. Then she presses her breasts against the wings of his scapulae, which she has called his angel wings. Closing his eyes, Aaron accepts Parvati's warmth and energy through his back, sending it on through his body into his palms. Within a few minutes, they hear the same soundscape that they have been hearing since he first used the instrument with her.

"What is it?" Niko asks.

"The sounds of our body and being as one entity."

Aaron details the low erratic tones of the gut, the rhythms of their heartbeats, the whooshes of their pulses, and the high-pitched whine of their bones. He concentrates on Vivaldi's *Four Seasons* and harmonizes the music of his body with hers and with that of Vivaldi.

When he has shown the others his mother and her consorts, Niko's friend Cistas, who is from a sister monastery in Samarkand, marvels at seeing and hearing the body transposed, and the monks wonder if they might use the instrument in their teaching. Niko remarks, "We might find a way for us to share more of the inner life with our pilgrims."

When the brothers and sisters have gone, Aaron moves his attention to the story that Parvati told him last week. His body shifts, and he can feel and hear that change in the music: The pitches flatten and resonate as minor and diminished chords. After a time, the rhythms of his body disarticulate, some elements quickening while others slow down. As they become arrhythmic, the soundscape smears like hands moving across wavy lines of fresh paint. He is fairly sure that rather than reaching an unfamiliar state of order, he is entering a greater level of disorder.

Aaron takes his hands off the wire mesh. After a pause, he gently lifts Parvati's hands to the instrument instead, whispering, "Play your cousins."

The soundscape she creates is at first unstable. It takes Aaron several minutes to make sense of it. Then he hears a sweet harmony come apart into a harsh noise that reminds him of a badly played organ. Reading his body carefully and vigilantly, he recognizes—with a lift that counters the heaviness of the soundscape—that the dysrhythmias and dissonances of her feelings are resonating with his in a way that is pulling his organ systems out of sync. He recognizes the feeling. He felt something similar when Leilani tried to control Sarah's mind, and again when he detected the dissolution of his DNA.

"That's it!" he exclaims. Aaron takes her palms and kisses each. Sudden quiet fills his ears and seems to stop his voice.

Parvati whispers, "You saw something?"

"I felt something. I felt the pattern of our dissonance, how you and I change over time, how this story pulled our states apart, and how our processes wove in and out of one another, converging and diverging through the instrument's harmonies and disharmonies. Every living community must experience this. Every community explores and elaborates its shared being in time, and each member encounters and influences the others. Syncing requires a strong shared state. It would have to be continuous."

"I think we've talked of it before," she says gently, not wishing to discourage him.

"Yes, but not as integral to the flesh. And there's something more. You're out of sync—your body is out of sync because of the tragedy of your cousins, and my body went along with it, but I couldn't make sense of it until I heard it. And then—then I recognized that the exquisite inner coordination of the flesh—which is synced in a complex way—was dysrhythmic. My organs were beginning to work against each other."

"You lost your rhythm?" she asks quizically.

"Not exactly. My rhythms went their separate ways. Your desire to weave the memory of your cousins back into your life is pulling you back in time while your desire to break the thread is pulling you forward. You're at odds within."

"Yes, of course."

"The community is doing the same thing. The restorationists are pulled back by the way things were and pulled forward by their vision of how things should be. Every guild sustains that kind of tension across time and builds a narrative that resolves it. The point is that the various elements of the community are going out of sync like the organs systems of a body that is failed by its inner union."

"And the habitat?" Parvati asks thoughtfully.

"Yes, I think so. The guilds are separate and out of sync inside and out—and so are their members. That could stress the body of humanity and its habitats—which adapt and evolve on different timescales."

"With Sarah's decline, every silken fiber of the subtle structure of our community may be slipping along every other. Our patterns are diverging"

"We can sync them in your body and see what we discover."

"Let's go beyond words this time—let's go back to music and dance."

Aaron smiles slyly. "We've drummed in and drummed out. Let's drum on."

Three weeks later, they return to the composer. They have tried grief work, paradox, saturnalia, yoga, classical Indian dance, pilgrimage walks, and many other rites and traditions, and have seen that they do not need help with release, which only weakens them; nor with exercise, which they prefer to enjoy in bed; nor with changing habits, of which only meals and sleep and conviviality remain. In fact, they wish to add a habit by playing the composer every few days, as it now and then reveals something new and potentially important.

This time, after they have observed Shabbat with Hebrew and Hindi blessings, and have retired to their chamber, Parvati says, "I would like to add an element to our Shabbat evenings—and to our everyday sessions. We, too, can bless this work."

She takes his hand and leads him to the bed, where they sit facing, and she says, "I invite us to be neither obedient nor disobedient; controlled nor controlling; superior nor inferior; slothful nor reactive; marred nor marring; corrupt nor pure; compliant nor defiant; codependent nor independent; anxious nor careless; with nor against; lagging nor leading."

"It's like Aristotle's virtue is the mean, or Maimonides' yetzer hatov, or a dynamic equilibrium. Wonderful."

"We should remember character as well as ethics."

"Yes. Amein."

She smiles lovingly, her gift well received. They are both happy.

Aaron says, "The beauty of your joy reminds me to share what I was thinking earlier today when you went to sit under your favorite cedar tree."

"What is it?"

"I've been looking back and down. I've embraced darkness. In a way, I've done that my whole life—before now. If I'm to find the unexpected, I should be looking above and ahead. I should be looking for time assets."

"Yes."

"You said as much the first week, didn't you?"

"I think it's a good idea," she says with a smile, "and I love sharing love and joy with you now, while I can."

He squeezes her hands tightly. "Okay to visit my dam and sires?"

She laughs. "Virtually, I presume?"

He laughs and kisses her dulce-de-leche neck, which seems to him to taste sweet, and goes to the composer to revisit the image of his mother and consorts that is always at the edge of his awareness. Seeing them all together, he reflects on the enactment, and with some effort brings each in turn to the foreground. Parvati looks at Aaron and at Dan, whose image is currently in focus, and says as if she is reading his mind, "Bloodline and God-wrestling time credits."

Aaron assents with a wordless exhalation of wonder. With effort, he brings Randall to the fore. Randall seems to give him a slight knowing grin. Aaron squeezes his eyelids shut; when he opens them again, the grin is gone. He wonders if he imagined it, or if it signals his subconscious embodiment of Randall or some kind of connection through Parvati or shared interbeing. With effort, he moves his mother and Randall side-by-side. Parvati laughs under her breath and says, "They both embodied the tree of life for the discovery of new knowledge. And formed a time credit."

Aaron gasps. "Yes! Do you recall how Randall did that during the enactment?"

"I wrote the actor's lines, but it was a guess. We don't know exactly how he embodied it."

"Well! Let's see if you come up with the same guess in union."

"I thought you'd never ask," she says playfully, but remains seated beside him on the floor, rapt. "Go on."

After a time, Aaron moves the image of John and the image of his mother close together. Abruptly, they age decades as Aaron's memory returns to his mother's last day in the hospice. He cannot see what it is that bound them, or what they shared that he might call an asset. He sighs tensely and says, "They solved problems together."

"They both had well-developed—if not wholly appreciated —character."

"They all did."

"True. But what exactly was it that enabled them to solve the problems that we saw them solve?"

"We can still ask."

"We must talk with John. He must come to us."

Aaron's heart swells, and he enters a sweet state of bright love. These antecedents illuminate the blanks in his vision that have impeded his being and becoming. He leaves a part of his awareness on the four figures and contemplates the luminous wall. The soundscape shifts; patterns seem to take shape in the fog, but they remain faint and abstract. They may be clues to his legacy, glimpses into the uncreated world. He does his best to enter the fog of unknowing and to find a way ahead.

He takes heart. Aaron begins to believe that he can sync with life in time, reach its moving front, and envision something of the future. He lets this state imprint his being so that he will be able to return to it, and to abide in it as they face the oppressive time debts. Then Aaron stops. The heaviness of grieving his mother and their lost innocence frightens him. He has always deflected it with understanding so as to preserve his heart, but this is the time when he must let it enter into his heart and abide there with the pain of losing all his childhood dreams. It will hurt more when they open Parvati's more traumatic disillusionment—but their joy in each other and their growing confidence in their third will ease it.

All week, they open their hearts to the body of life and explore possible embodiments of the tree of life, which Parvati melds with tantric practices that graft the tree onto the trunk of the energy body. They begin with upward ascents to the unformed potentials above their heads that they then draw down into their heart centers, and farther down into the earth to join heaven and earth. They invite the eternal to manifest in the real. By the next Sabbath, they have rooted the Judaic tree in the heart, and placed the top of the tree above their crowns, where their joined focus can easily ascend to it. They then pattern the descent of new apprehension and comprehension to the eye of the heart, and then down the central channel through the root chakra into the ground.

On that Sabbath, they welcome John with a shared bear hug that includes Gina, Lena, and Lisa. They enjoy a rather intense dinner together, after which Gina and her wives go to teach fertility in the forest theater. A group of Niko's friends takes John out to show him the climbing wall and rappelling generator, and he has the pleasure of watching them use some of the route-setting ideas that he learned when he and his son enjoyed trad and bouldering.

The window-rattling winds of late fall dissuade them from venturing into the forest, where boughs may break. Parvati does not mind in the least when Aaron and John choose the indoor tropical dining area for a late drink and snack and kibitzing session that grows serious and—for Aaron and John—both complicated and motivated by their memories of Melissa.

"We saw the enactment, for which you gave me so much kind assistance," says Parvati, "but in getting to know Aaron I have in some ways lost the big picture. Your perspective is key now as we engage time assets from Melissa and her consorts. We have identified what we think are the central ones that derive from her work with Randall and Dan, but we cannot see how you solved problems with her, and what time assets we may be able to draw on as we try to do the same."

"Ah! I see," John replies. "Well … I don't know. It came naturally. We didn't analyze it then—and of course we wouldn't have analyzed it then as we might do now."

Aaron asks, "Can you recall what you relied on her for, or welcomed most from her?"

"Let me ask this first: What do you have so far?"

Parvati explains. John gives her a look of perfect incomprehension and says didactically, "So you are still developing your methods, and have yet to form the legacy."

Parvati looks at Aaron, who smiles and says to John, "Now you do sound like Mom. But that was then and this is now, and we're preparing to form our offering."

Parvati slumps comically in her chair. "My dear John, you make it sound as if we haven't even started!"

"I do? Or it's true?"

Parvati and Aaron gaze at each other. After a long minute, he says, "Our third has yet to go supernova."

John looks puzzled. "So ... your mom and I ... had a third?"

"Many!" Parvati says.

"We solved a problem, but—"

"Yes, just so. And we'd like to solve one, too, and could use some clues from you as to how you two worked together."

"Like two halves of one soul."

"Yes. How?"

John has never broken it down. It takes some time, and many questions, to get John to think differently about his interaction with Melissa. At last it becomes easy. "Well," he says, "she was the one who immersed herself in what was happening on the ground, so to speak—or under and above ground, to be more precise. She was, I suppose, earthy, practical, empirical, and systematic."

"And you?"

"I had a broad fund of knowledge of all kinds—broad bandwidth as we used to call it. And I drew from many sources of frames and constructs when forming a solution. I could improvise across styles without losing the melody."

"So ... she was chords and theme and you were melody?"

John's eyebrows go up. "She was structure and I was improv."

Aaron looks at Parvati, who smiles and raises her eyebrows. "Can you teach Parvati to improvise? I'm the earth-bound one."

"Everyone knows how. You play the rate and rhythm and colors of your heart."

The next week, Parvati comes into the room looking for Aaron. He is walking in a line, making a pattern with his feet.

"Another pattern."

"Yes! After this we'll probably have all the patterns we need, and will be ready to contemplate our third—as a vision."

"An image?"

"A vision of the future, a New World derived from this one—in the context of the community, that is."

Parvati teases, "And how long will we be here?"

"Given the way I feel here, with you, I hope it's forever." He jogs over and takes her hand. "Let's say our vision is straight ahead, on the wall."

"An image."

"A portal. We want to see it, to get closer. When it turns out to be a mirage, we envision another beyond the first."

She begins to lead him toward it.

"Wait," he laughs. "We have to know where we are."

"And where is that?"

"Well, behind us is the life experience that formed our priming and our stances, which impel us and direct us toward our vision."

"This is your mother's pattern! Remind me what primes it?"

"The events—good and bad—that motivate us."

"Okay. Anything else?"

"Yes. With our debts pushing us, and the vision beyond the portal pulling us, we use our assets to form our stance and to devise strategies and skills. Can you embody that?"

"Yes. And I harness that to what state?"

"Fertile care."

"Of course. And now?"

"And now we identify the strategies and skills that will get us there—and then go there."

"I hope we're past the character-forming part," she smiles.

"No more falls, please!"

"I think we're ready for the vision, strategies and skills," Aaron assures.

Parvati leads Aaron by the hand to the opposite wall. "Our vision is on the other side," she teases.

"After you," he teases back.

13

Kindred

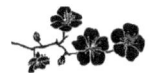

The first procession of initiates arrives from the lodge, enters the main door of the forest sanctuary, and approaches the altar. Rafa, Mitzi, and Yuko-Hyun direct them to form a circle broken by seven aisles, and to form more concentric circles behind the first. Parvati can feel the room filling with fertile care states, and asks Aaron if she should pattern them with the transformative state now. She listens for an answer, but hears no reply. She is beginning to think that she never will, and that he was right about his body creating his being through its record of his ephemeral experience. His unique body and its record of life on earth may be gone for good.

Fortunately, like his mother, Aaron put his all into the whole and so—but for his flesh—is wholly available to her. He is still here in her, and in this part of the body of humanity and is lifting her spirits for this day of joyful renewal. She and the others will transmit his last and best gifts to those here who work ceaselessly to restore and sustain God-evolved life. She need not speak of his sacrifice as if death were his third; she will not remember him as a reason for sorrow or defeat. She will keep to the purpose that gave meaning to his last days, and to all his days.

Parvati watches the procession of initiates who live away, glad that those traveling with the Green School or stationed in remote habitats have returned for the fulfillment of this legacy, which promises to change their way of life for the better. As the fabro guilders begin to file in, Dirk pushes past them and strides to the center to ask, "Is Aaron still alive?"

Rafa turns to Parvati and, seeing her consternation, realizes that she has made a mistake. "*Tío* never said not to say he was sick."

Parvati's carefully composed manner crumbles, and she glances at Björn. He has been her rock, but he, too, has been sad since she told him that Aaron was sick, and has been grieving since the monks interred Aaron in their subterranean catacomb. Even so, Björn has stepped up as able, and she has taken Aaron's advice to heart and turned to Björn more and more in her time of need.

John steps in, saying smoothly, "Aaron didn't want his limitations to become ours, or to let the imprint of illness and death mark or mar the rite. Since you ask, we can say that the monks put him to rest yesterday."

Dirk nods. Everyone sitting close to the center heard, and passes the information on to the back. Parvati sees that she must say something, and her confidence wavers. An unexpected gust of wind tousles nearby treetops, spraying the procession with icy darts of sweet water. She puts aside dark thoughts and signals her former students to create their transformative states, which are like cure states. These spread rapidly and prime the room with anticipation, determination, and daring.

When all are seated, either in the sanctuary or outside under the tent-like membrane extension, Parvati walks around the inner circle of participants, pausing between aisles to speak to those in each section. "As most of you now know, Aaron died two nights ago. He had wanted to join us in body, but death took him, and it will be up to us who loved him to bring him to life again through his legacy. His last wish was that you would focus on the rite, and over the next few days give yourself to its truth for each and all. After the rite, any of you who wish to observe Aaron's passing are invited to come to the family memorial tomorrow at noon."

Parvati pauses to look out at the steady rain that filters down the fir needles, filling both the spongy soil and their lungs with the water of life. She comes to herself only after the others in the center have opened the trap doors, set up a seven-sided altar, and shepherded the community's new life—human and otherwise— inside to the center to crawl or to sit and play. She had planned to ask those who did not have young ones to bring artifacts to the center and place them on the altar, but the room is so well primed that she skips ahead to say, "Take a moment to look at the thirds in the center who represent our future, and who motivate our community, and to hold up the those artifacts that represent the rest of your thirds."

Parvati notices that Cookie raises an image of his burnt habitat, Siobhan one of Leilani, and others hold remembrances of things they would change. One has raised up an image of the betweeners; another of the island where they exile malefactors; a third of fear addicts they turned away; a fourth of the coyote pack that bypassed the monitors; and many others hold images of poison barrens, fire barrens, sand lines, and new dunes. If the sync eases their work and frees energy, they may be able to act on these.

Parvati takes heart and nods to Oke Ten, who walks with ceremony from the center up to the huge gong that dangles from a frame positioned inside the wall. He takes the cloth-covered mallet from the frame and strikes the gong. An infant and a lamb cry; a turkey escapes its caretaker. Sarah laughs suddenly and says, "See how the rain is easing, and hear the birds herald the day. Take this daybreak as a sign that we are embarking on a new life!"

Sarah takes Parvati's arm and guides her around the circle as the others at the center lead the young outside and disassemble and stow the altar. After a time, she nudges Parvati, who begins to speak. "Today we will reconcile a shared time debt: the loss of momentum and synchronization. This debt has arisen from our ways of life, which have become disjointed and fixed and are impeding our progress and disengaging our motion from our action. To put it plainly, we have gotten in our own way, and it is time we moved on more freely."

Sarah continues, "We will begin by forming a new guild called the Alguild for habitat representation. This will be the umbrella guild, the guild of all guilds. It will hold others so that each guild can open its boundaries to all who wish to gain or contribute knowledge that furthers the guild's purpose."

In place of the expected roar, Parvati hears stunned silence; she continues. "When we have formed the Alguild, we will enact a dance to break old social patterns and form new ones. The guild and dance will constitute the first annual synchronization rite, which we will all reenact on the shortest day of every year until the time when we are privileged to repattern it anew."

Sarah says, "As always, each of us will be responsible for our own faith in life, and for constructing meaning and purpose that harmonize our shared interbeing. Now, we will be restructuring this interbeing and reintegrating with it in this rite so as to synchronize more closely with the moving front of time."

Parvati announces, "We will now choose the first seven

Alguild elders. All circles now join hands." Rafa and Yuko-Hyun show the bewildered folk in the front row what to do. Those behind them imitate the front row.

Parvati smiles at their surprise, and says, "All stand, still holding hands. Now, at the sound of the gong, the front row will shuffle-step very slowly to the right in time with the drum until you are revolving slowly and steadily around the center. Second row, you begin on the next gong, third row on the third gong, and so on to the last row."

Parvati signals Oke Ten to sound the gong. The drummer beside him takes up a slow and steady beat on the bodhrán to guide the shuffling feet. Rafa and Yuko-Hyun help the inner circle close gaps between those who took hands across an aisle and to open breathing space between those who are pressed together. Before the second gong sounds, the first row is well-spaced and moving smoothly. The rows are added in turn until each person in each row is stepping in unison, and the inner circle has completed many revolutions while the outer circle has made only half of one revolution.

"Stop!" Parvati calls. The drum goes silent. "Front row, reform your aisles."

One person from the center goes to the place of each aisle and holds an arm out to show where the new aisle will be. Rafa and Yuko-Hyun help them to bring those in between the aisles together so as to create new aisles. With coaching, the community forms seven aisles that extend from the front row to the back.

"Yes! Good." Sarah says, holding her hands palms-upward, "You have just formed seven palms."

Parvati moves to the group of people between the aisles closest to her and says, "You who form this palm will hold the forest habitat. You will support your randomly-chosen elder in forming the first Alguild after this first annual synchro rite."

"The forest habitat is the largest," says a voice. "Shouldn't we have more than one elder?"

"As we all know, no habitat can exist without all the others, thus each palm will carry equal weight in dialogue and decision-making."

"And unequal responsibility."

Sarah says, "No. This is for representation, not for the physical work of restoration."

Parvati goes to each of the remaining six palms in turn and tells them that they will be holding saltwater, littoral, field, wetland, sweet water, or "other" habitats. Then she says, "Each palm will sustain its share of the ongoing dialogue of the whole, raise concerns—especially those related to the habitat or habitats they hold—and co-lead exploration of dynamic equilibria and change."

Sarah continues, "The purpose of the Althing is to join each of us with all of life in time. This year, the Althing will examine our synchronization of being and interbeing with the body of life in time and discern old habits that are in the way. It will be up to the palms to do the real work of observing your habitat, detecting problems and possibilities, and responding with personal changes in the moment or by raising concerns with your guild elder to take to the quarterly meetings of the guild of the whole. This guild will bring your work into the dynamic process of adaptive transformation initiated by Aaron's legacy transmission."

Parvati adds, "This rite will support us in changing the way we change, until we are able to change continuously and without representation."

Sarah interjects with a laugh, "Which may take a very long time!"

Parvati smiles and continues, her heart lightened by the sight of Aaron's legacy—and hers—coming to life. "We still hold the historic habit of drawing lines around what belongs to us and what does not. Even here, where we recognize the continuity of life in time, we say to ourselves, I'm responsible for this and not for that. In this rite, we become more aware of these habits so that we can own and change them as we go. We will draw any lines as if we were drawing them on the shore at low tide, where the tide will wash them away."

Sarah says, "This year, the Alguild will place special emphasis on entering into a broad and rich and deep and fluid dialogue that will lead to sync, and that will never repeat. If the sync does not happen easily, there are unseen obstacles. Each member of each palm will look out for unrecognized patterns, search for unseen gaps, and patiently and persistently engage the known and penetrate the unknown. When you raise a concern, and an individual or group response is not enough to resolve it, own it. Raise it with everyone you can until it is resolved or bring it to your elder, who will bring it to the Alguild."

Parvati continues, "This is the way that each of you becomes part of the palm for which your elder will speak. For the elders, the Alguild will be a crucible to hold transformative states like those you are feeling here, now. These may prime elders to conduct impassioned dialogue, to destroy obstacles to accord, to vaporize sterile rumination, and to otherwise cure ills that bar the community from finding the best way forward in continuity, adaptation, and deep change of all as one. To do otherwise is to sustain uncoupled motions until we all wind down."

Hands go up. Sarahs says, "Please hold your questions until we have chosen one elder to be held by each palm."

Björn opens a trap door in the center and hoists out a large box. Removing the lid, he lifts the box up out of Parvati's sightline but within her reach. The drum rolls. She reaches in, retrieves a piece of paper, unfolds it, and reads, "The elder for forest is ... Neli Rakasanayan."

A timid young woman of small stature stands from the back row. She opens her eyes wide, folds her arms, and shakes her head. Parvati suppresses a smile. Neli is a schooler who has almost earned initiation, but appears much younger than many of her peers. Parvati feels life energy flow to her palms, but is too far away to share love with a student in that way, so she allows her voice to fill with love instead as she says, "Neli, this year the forest palm will hold you while you finish your studies."

"What if I don't want to?" she chirps dubiously. "Or can't?"

A voice from the forest palm group speaks up, saying, "We want you to!"

"Yes!" cry several others.

An elderly voice adds, "Better a young voice than an old one!"

Another says, "The palm will do the work, the elder will give it voice."

"You should have someone who knows more," Neli says dubiously.

"You know all of us," comes the reply.

She shrugs, "I can try."

The palm applauds. When the noise dies down, Sarah says, "Does the forest palm vow to support its elder by engaging in dialogue about synchro that she can bring to the dialogue of the whole; by raising concerns that pertain to your habitat; and by exploring the unperceived, unseen, and unknown?"

"Yes!" respond a few clear voices.

"Everyone say yes, or say why!" Sarah admonishes with a wry smile.

"Yes!"

Parvati says, "Neli, you should know that after the first year, you will continue to serve on the Althing as a retiring elder. After that, you will be ineligible to serve again for fourteen years."

Neli shrugs again with raised eyebrows and plops back down. The sanctuary falls silent. The rain has stopped, but the wind shakes the branches above the sanctuary, releasing waves of falling water. Parvati signals Björn, who raises the box again. She selects another name and calls, "The elder for saltwater is Sam Celery."

Sam Celery stands and opens his fried-egg eyes wide. He laughs through the wide gaps between his front teeth and takes a comical bow. Parvati recognizes Sam as a prickly eccentric known for never having cut his long white hair, for wearing seal-skin clothes that he makes himself, and for playing his banjo so fast and loud that he is always in conflict with his neighbors in the tree houses. Sam arrived here late in life from a place Parvati can't remember.

Parvati fills with doubt. She has been counting on selecting charismatic or winsome or earnest leaders who can hold the unarticulated hopes and dreams of others. She is not sure that Sam can do this. She and Aaron talked of the size of the guild; they recognized that a small one might become unstable and fail while a large one might become unwieldy and fall into factions. They had decided to err on the side of caution by selecting another round of elders should the first seem unpromising. She does not want to be a source of doubt, but if doubt arises she will address it now, when she can.

Parvati chooses the next sheet of paper and reads the name from it with relief and anticipation. "The elder for littoral will be ... Miriam Price."

Miriam waves. Miriam is a big woman who sits in the common room after dinner and tells stories to children who gather in her lap and around her knees. She reminds Parvati of a storyteller figurine that Aaron's mother gave to him, and that he passed on to her when he entrusted her with their legacy. Miriam is fond of everyone and everyone—especially the very young or very old—is fond of her. She will mentor Neli and bring out the best in Sam.

Parvati selects another paper. "The elder for field is Takes Ten Paces."

Paces is a thirty-something fine art guilder with a long braid who speaks sparingly and laughs rarely, and yet his intense personal magnetism draws everyone within forty meters of his core. Paces has not a drop of indigenous blood, but has studied many forms of esoteric personal transformation, and has taken the spirit of One Crazy Raven for his root guru. He has progressed beyond all his peers and elders in the most stringent Shamanic training, which she suspects he may be using as a complex-any. Paces could easily dominate the new guild, but would never do so. He seems unhappy to be chosen, but she knows that she can count on him to serve his palm well. Parvati smiles inwardly. She would like to be a fly on the wall during the first meeting of this unexpected group.

Parvati selects another paper. "The elder for wetland is ... Bailey Nagy."

Everyone knows her; she is impossible to avoid. Bailey belongs to the performance guild and is always embodying and performing new or favorite characters at dinnertime. Her favorite is the Hungarian woman who speaks English with a heavy accent and wears the antique folk skirts that Bailey found in her father's ancestral village. She is so beautiful and charismatic and sexually expressive that she has taken two consorts and is rumored to be courting a third. If her persona dominated the council, it would become a party. Fortunately, this group is too strong to accept the role of audience.

Parvati says with a smile, "The elder for sweet water is … Kim Coltrane."

Parvati couldn't be more pleased. Kim has been privy to Aaron's reasoning and integral to the creation of the rite; she will be able to transmit more than Parvati could tell the Alguild about the legacy—if they were to ask. And she knows that Kim will know when to consult Sarah or Doug or John. Fortune is smiling on this Alguild, and Parvati is grateful for it.

Parvati reads the next name, "The elder for other is … Ceta Matsutake."

This skeleton-thin woman grew up with mycologist parents and is dedicated—apparently to an unhealthy degree—to photography and digital recording. She lives like a renunciate and avoids others except to look at them and record them through lenses. Parvati expects that joining the Althing will transform Ceta, who will take it seriously and break through her constraints.

"What is other?" Ceta asks with a frown.

Parvati replies, "Other includes built habitats like human lodges and animal burrows; extreme environments like rocky crags, caves, and burns; and modified habitats, including outdoor and indoor agro, which will soon include plantings in the lodge and other non-purpose-built structures. Your palm will have to devote time this year to working with the agro and restoration guilds to catalogue and classify local and satellite habitats."

"We can use photos. And look at habitats built by other species, like plants that emit chemicals toxic to their neighbors."

"Excellent work, Ceta! You can gather everything and anything not belonging to others. You've already begun."

Sarah says, "Now let's take time to refresh our bodies and let this settle and raise concerns. We will reconvene in twenty minutes for discussion of the whole."

As the group disbands, Parvati pulls Sarah aside. "I'd like a little time for myself, but I don't want to run off if you need me."

Sarah embraces her, and Parvati realizes that they have not hugged for a long time. Sarah whispers in her ear, "Thank you so much. That was wonderful. The body of the community can take it from here. They should. They must."

"Don't worry. I may not be in the building, but I'll be here."

"You aren't ready to go out into the world and bring more of it into your story. Not yet. But you will."

"Are you asking me to leave?"

"No! Don't go before I do, or before they're ready." Sarah begins to cry.

"*Satch*! You can count on me to stay through the transitions."

Releasing Parvati, but still holding her arm with one hand, Sarah calls to Rafa, "Let's do the dance tonight, downstairs."

"That would ... that would be better," Rafa agrees. "The dry and wet suits went fast, and we just put a lot of work in front of us."

Parvati says, "Good idea. The cold and wet of the low tide zone would only distract the dancers."

Sarah's face contracts for a moment. She looks a century older. Lifting her robes, she releases Parvati's arm. "I miss him, too. See you at dinner."

∾

Sarah, Doug, and John are seated in a corner of the dance room on ceremonial cushions that Björn placed on a high platform.

"I'm glad Björn set up this platform," Sarah remarks.

"He's half performance guilder. I wish I could see. My night vision is getting worse and worse," Doug complains.

"Along with your nose hairs."

"Don't get me started on your sagging boobs."

"Nonsense. We're perfect for each other!"

John laughs. There is a bit of an edge in his tone.

"What?" Doug demands.

"I can't believe you guys only just figured that out."

"It was the S & M. Can't recommend it," Doug replies.

"It was bad timing," John disagrees. "I'm the expert on that. But there's nothing in your way now."

Doug sighs. "Yeah. I guess we shouldn't wait for one of us to croak."

Sarah says, "The stakes are as low as they're going to get."

"There's an argument against good timing," John puts in with a shake of the head.

"Ah, hell with it. I'm sick of playing Devil's Advocate. Let's just say that dark consorts are consorts, too, and when they run through their shit their dark stuff is all behind them."

"Are you talking about retirement?" Sarah asks ironically.

"I'm talking about I'd like you to keep me warm at night."

"Can you rephrase that?"

"Be my wife?"

"Host a wedding? That could fly. But I'd want to sleep in twin beds."

"Like the couples in those television shows that raised us," John teases.

"Like all that shit we can't forget," Doug curses amiably.

"Promise me you'll curse-bless me every day?" Sarah asks Doug. "I could use the spice. As I get older everything gets blander—even life and death."

Doug gripes amiably, "How long is this thing gonna go on?"

John ignores Doug. "This is the happiest and most alive I've ever been. I never thought all that would come to me through you, Sarah."

"Oh, God. I was awful. I knew everything."

"Even Doug remembers that."

"I was always watching you. But you were too smart to waste energy keeping track of me."

"Okay, let's cut the sugar," Doug says, gesturing toward the dancers. "If we have to stay, tell me what's going on. They look like they're playing a dozen games of rugby."

"They're enacting the old pattern of vocation. Each of those scrums is a guild, and the guild members are facing inward, defending the center; the ones running around them are initiates trying to get in. Once everyone gets in, the guilds hold them in unless they manage to escape. If a lot escape, this phase of the dance could go on for quite a while! If not, it will fade into the next phase in which the guild elders face outward and form a core, and the members and initiates form patterns by moving around them."

"Old pattern, new pattern?" John asks.

"Just so," Sarah replies.

"How many phases are there?" Doug whines.

"They're dancing birth, maturation, initiation, vocation,

lifework, legacy transmission, legacy work, and death."

"No afterlife?" Doug teases.

"We leave that to the individual," Sarah says. "As the religious science folk used to say, if we were supposed to know about it, we would."

"So, we're halfway there?" John asks.

"Not really. Lifework and legacy work are very long."

"Aaron's wasn't."

"Most people work on theirs alone; his was a community effort. We had to join together to pick up the threads you and Melissa broke," Sarah says.

"Sorry," John replies.

"Don't be. Your work was a great blessing to the Age of Life in Time."

After a long pause, during which the three old friends watch the rite, John muses, "I like this. I never appreciated dance, but this is allowing us to see and feel the problem as Aaron did, and to see his solution too."

"His and Parvati's."

"Go on, say it," Doug says. "We all wish Aaron was here to see it."

"We're so lucky he reached completion. It was too much to expect, of course, but he has a lot of his mother in him—and had Parvati, too."

"Had a lot of his mother in him," John corrects sadly.

"As does Rafa. It's like Missy's still here," Sarah remarks.

"Better. Missy could get grumpy!" Doug counters.

"It's too soon to be gossiping about them like this!" John declares.

"Not at all," Doug says. "This is the beginning of their wake."

"We have to gossip while we can," Sarah adds, ironically.

"But if all three of us start talking about Missy, we'll sound like note jazz; we'll carry three parallel story lines that go on about who she was, as if she was three different people."

"Stories are simple," Doug points out. "Life is complex."

"That's how it is," Sarah says. "What we have of Missy today is what she was—and is—to each of us and to everyone else entangled with her. You know, Rafa is going to multiply that entanglement here by getting the teams that staff her clinics to found a Cure Guild to diagnose, treat, and cure diseases of habitats."

John looks envious. "That's going to get interesting, really interesting. I hope I hang around long enough to see that."

"We hope so, too. We need someone to gossip with," Doug teases.

John continues, "This change in interbeing, this ability to hold transformative states like cure states, is bringing this place alive."

"I hate to admit it," Sarah says, "but I agree. We focused too much on being at the cost of doing. We nurtured when we should have taken hard decisions."

"That approach suits restoration. You're moving on to habitat interception, which means it's time to create a more varied and complex way of life."

Sarah puts her hand on Doug's knee and looks across Doug to John. "We're about to live the next wrench, aren't we? We lived the one that started when Reggie shared her visualization, and this one will catch us unawares, too—even though we have our eyes open and see it coming."

"Change is change, and it's coming fast and free—which is a good sign."

"I think we're going to make it as a species," Doug says.

John and Sarah exchange looks.

"What?"

"You really are done being Devil's Advocate," John says with a wry smile.

"Don't look for him," Doug replies. "Aaron took him out."

"And Parvati."

"And you," Doug says. He puts his arm around Sarah, she rests her head on his shoulder, John puts an arm around both of them, and the three old friends watch the rite to the end before going to sleep in Sarah's room.

Acknowledgments

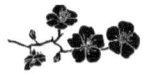

I would like to thank for my faith in a living future and in creating better character, better lives, and a better future: Maimonides and the *yetzer hara-yetzer hatov* practice; Samuel Sewall and his fellow Puritans; Benjamin Franklin; the DIY, self-help, and localist movements; and Thomas More's *Utopia*, the Prophets, *Star Trek*, Paul Hawken, Alice Walker, Paul Rogat Loeb, and the Age-ing to Sage-ing and Compassionate Cities movements.

Secondly, I am indebted for my confidence in the species to the wise continuation by indigenous peoples of their past care of life; to Christian communities that arose in the wake of the Roman Empire in France and elsewhere; to the communities that have practiced right living in North America, especially the Ebenezer Colony that continues as the Amanas in Iowa; as well as to the Mormons, Mennonites, Amish, New Hasidim, and New Monastics who support a living future.

Thirdly, I owe my inspiration to the new era that is already emerging. Examples include: the localist organic economy in Bow-Edison; the many examples given by Paul Hawken in *Blessed Unrest*; Puget Consumer Cooperative and the food co-op movement; Natural Grocers; the Living Futures Institute; the Bullitt Center; Greystone Publishing; builders of cob houses in the Lower Gulf Islands of British Columbia; Earthship Biotecture and the building of earthships around the world; and in Seattle

Earthcorps and in Southern Oregon: Lomakatsi, KS Wild, Coyote Trails, and Southern Oregon Land Conservancy—and the Pacific Northwest chapter of the Society for Ecological Restoration.

On a more personal note, I wish to thank my mother and her Swedish-American community, which taught that God is love, and that imbued a practical, capable, and responsible ethos of service to the greater good. I would also like to thank the Swedish relations who remain at Korndahl for showing us the farm the family has sustained for over 500 years, and that is part arable and pasture and part forested wetland.

Last and not least, I am grateful to the Southern Oregon team that made this book beautiful. The appearance is due to the professional competence and creativity of cover artist Bruce Bayard and book designer Chris Molé. The readability is due mainly to coach Chansonette Buck and editors Deidre Krupp, Deborah Mokma, and Ann DiSalvo.

Such writing ability as I am developing, I owe first to my father, who taught me reading and writing at a young age. I am also grateful to editor friends Eva Silverfine and Stephanie Holt for their talent and skill in verbal expression, to writing teacher Andrea Goldsmith of the Victorian Writer's Centre, and to Wendy Call of Hugo House. They kindly put up with an unusual and neurotoxic student, trusting that their wisdom would not go to waste.

Thank you also to my book development and beta readers, especially: Jan Agosti, Anna Barón, Jessica Bondy, Cynthia Bradley, Julie Clayton, Stephanie Holt, Christopher Howell, Joel Mason, Sara Myers Wade, Berta Nicol-Blades, and Dana Smaller. Special thanks to Jan, Anna, Julie, and Stephanie for their kindness in dark times.

About the Author

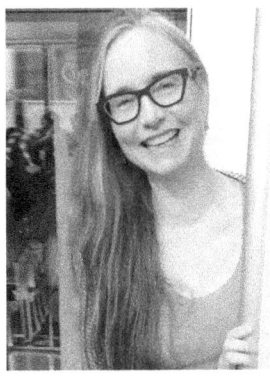

Beth Alderman, MD, MPH earned her AB and MD degrees from the University of Chicago and her MPH from the University of Washington. After Board Certification in Preventive Medicine and Public Health, she took a faculty position in the University of Colorado Medical School Department of Preventive Medicine, Biometrics, and Medical Informatics, where she did population-based epidemiological studies of adverse reproductive outcomes and methodological studies in clinical epidemiology. In her next faculty position at the University of Washington School of Public Health, she focused on risk factors for birth defects.

In 1996, she fell ill with the mysterious new plague and was given the provisional diagnosis "chronic fatigue syndrome". She has spent her time since studying her own case and pondering the reasons that her beloved profession failed her so completely. Fortunately, she discovered her cure, which may be of use to others suffering from one or more of the emerging epidemics affecting humans, their habitats, and life on earth.

For more about and from the author, see the following websites:

BethAldermanMD.com	*Free Information for all readers*
DoctorsOfLife.com	*For care and cure of all lives as one*
LivingFutureBooks.com	*Publishing Website*
LivingFutureCourses.com	*Educational Website with Free and advanced Courses*

Look for author's books on Amazon.com

Other Books by
Beth Alderman

Medical Phenomenology:
Chronic Ambient Poisoning
ISBN: 978-1-7332849-2-9

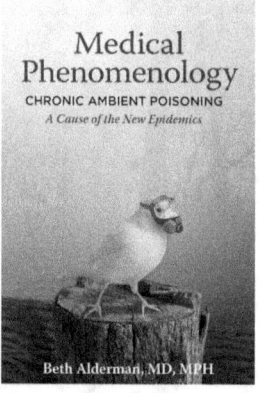

One day in December of 1996, the author (a physician, medical detective, and academic epidemiologist) developed disabling brain fog following on a decade-long descent into a painful, pervasive, and unprecedented chronic illness. Having done population-based studies to research the causes of birth defects, and having thus encountered the limitations of modern methods, she had inadvertently prepared to investigate the causes of her illness—which was given the provisional and uninformative label of "chronic fatigue."

The author began a delineation of the natural history of her condition using the methods of: doctors Hippocrates, Maimonides and Oliver Sacks; the "radical empiricism" used by Dr. William James; and the phenomenology introduced by Teilhard de Chardin and Merleau-Ponty. After a fifteen-year search, she found a doctor of integrative medicine whose elimination diet relieved her brain fog, which enabled her to complete a self-study and to construct an actionable new diagnosis: chronic ambient poisoning. Unseen by doctors and obscured by medical dogma and a myriad of false diagnoses, chronic ambient poisoning defies late modern, fragmented, accuracy-challenged medical research methods and delivery systems. It also reveals that human-caused habitat injuries that afflict birds, bees, and other species are affecting humans while driving evolved life toward extinction in the way of an asteroid strike. To ignore this diagnosis is to ignore the dangers to all lives posed by maladaptive modern lifeways.

The Evolve Fertility Series

BOOK 1
Melissa's Match: *Great Society*
ISBN: 978-1-7321110-1-1

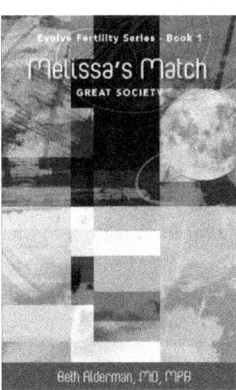

It's the early 1970s. Melissa and her friends begin their first year of college in the inner city of Chicago at a time when post-assassination riots, Great Society scholarship programs, and veterans returning from Vietnam create a sometimes explosive confluence of urban and rural, rich and poor, white and black, educated and uneducated. Coming of age in a violent, unjust, and yet hopeful time, they struggle to reconcile their hopes and opportunities with the shadows of war and the destructive clashes of senescing and emerging systems of care and cure of life on earth.

BOOK 2
Connie's Conception: *Awareness of Peril*
ISBN: 978-1-7321110-0-4

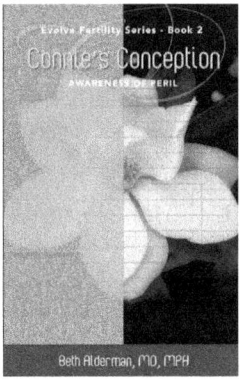

It's the late 1980s, and Connie Martin, a doctor working for the Epidemiology Intelligence Service of the CDC, is called to Colorado to investigate an alarming outbreak of birth defects. Born illegitimate in the San Luis Valley as Consuela Martín, a name known only to close friends and to her beloved gamer and programmer husband, she arrives as an unknown. Joined by environmental activists who suspect the state's Superfund sites and by doctors and parents who fear for its children, Connie attempts to discover the link between habitat destruction and damage to innocents.

BOOK 3
Melissa's Malady: *End of Modernity*
ISBN: 978-1-7321110-2-8

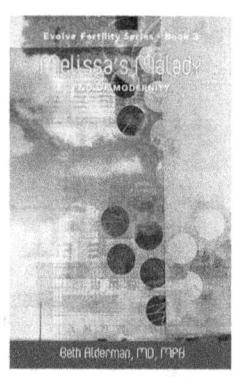

IIt is almost the year of the millennium, and Melissa meets her college friends Sarah and Doug and her first and only true love John for a reunion in Hyde Park. All four are in the midst of their careers. All struggle with the compromises that have marred their happiness. All wish to change the world, each in a different way. Sarah has left her government job for a new life as a yoga teacher. Doug is helping to birth a new value-based economy. John is a successful academic doctor. Melissa is ailing. They unite to turn John's success as a researcher to the cure of Melissa's mysterious chronic illness. What they find will change their lives and their imperiled world.

BOOK 4
Colette's Creativity: *Sacred and Profane*
ISBN: 978-1-7321110-3-5

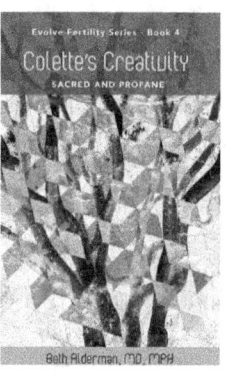

Colette, Melissa's childhood friend, abandons her marriage and home in Maine and flies to Melbourne. There she is taken in by her friend Reggie, who seems to know the secret of joy. Colette joins in the lives of striking individuals who lead her to view sexuality as a manifestation of the sacred. As she leaves behind the wounds caused by profane sexuality, she and her new friends clash with members of Reggie's family who force them to flee and to begin again.

BOOK 5
Colette's Community: *Thirds*
ISBN: 978-1-7321110-4-2

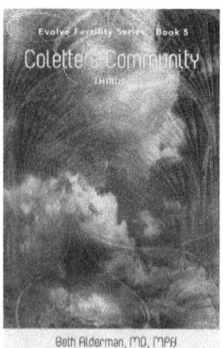

Soon after Colette and her friends find a new home, an old boyfriend of Melissa's who is sojourning in Australia calls and expresses his desire to visit. Colette plans to use the visit as a chance to develop a job for herself; he plans to check up on Colette for Melissa. As they get to know each other, they see that despite differences in religion, origin, and experience, they are on very similar spiritual paths. When it is time for Randall to go home, Colette joins him in Chicago. When he becomes caught up in his old life, however, she returns to Australia to pursue her dream of giving birth to a sacred community.

Chronic Illness Owner's Manuals
Regenerate Your Life: Chronic Illness as a Springboard for Creating Your Best Life

ISBN: 978-1-7321110-8-0 (VOL. 1)

ISBN: 978-1-7321110-9-7 (VOL. 2)

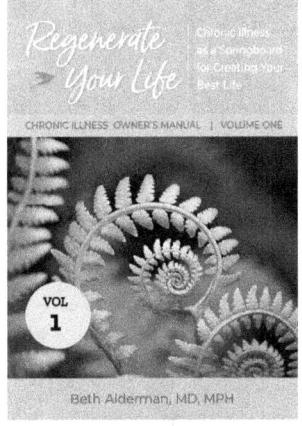

The *Chronic Illness Owner's Manual* series is for patients with chronic illness, and for the people who care for them. Suitable for individual or small group use, it offers a comprehensive, systematic, step-by-step approach to engaging modern medical systems, and to healing from the inside out.

The books comprise anecdotes, exercises, and quotes that address recovery through seven aspects of the body: awareness, understanding, perceptions, sensations, energy, flesh, and interbeing. The frames, constructs, patterns, and processes employed by the series are drawn from traditions of medicine, field biology, theology, and psychology from around the globe. Their synthesis offers an emerging, sustainable, eco-centric, eco-contextual, and customizable approach to creating a new and better life that regenerates your unique meaning, purpose, and vision of abundant life. The *Chronic Illness Owner's Manual* series complements care and cure courses available online at www.LivingFutureCourses.com.

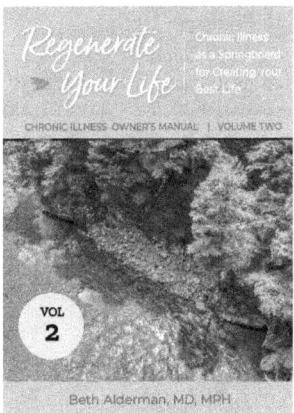

The Evolve Restoration Series
Sequel to the Evolve Fertility Series

BOOK 1
Pilgrim Minds: *After the War on Life*

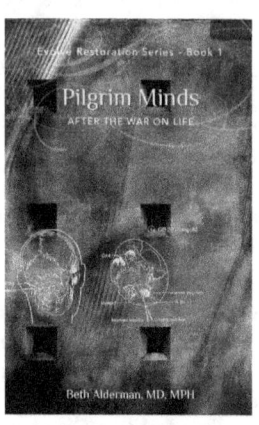

ISBN: 978-1-7321110-5-9

Melissa's deathbed request catapults her son Aaron on a journey from her family's Mississippian clinic to the Salish Sea to claim a mysterious legacy. Meeting his niece Rafa en route, he continues overland with her, and uncle and niece come to know and depend on each other. On arriving at the Saltspring Island Research Center (SIRC), Sarah, now the keeper of the center's narratives, confesses that Aaron's legacy is a task: to apply his mother's philosophy to SIRC's lifeways in order to revitalize it.

While he had been immersed in his mother's medical philosophy, SIRC had used many of her ideas to found a fertility school. SIRC's encroaching apathy persuaded Sarah that they missed one or more essential lifeways, and hopes that Aaron may be able to pinpoint and provide them. Taken by surprise, but ready to step up, Aaron immerses himself in the community, and Rafa undergoes SIRC's initiation process. Uncle and niece come to love Cascadia and to relish local, burgeoning patterns of innovation. Both choose to stay at SIRC, an agentic community that is doing much to restore evolution and its living future.

BOOK 2
Aaron's Legacy: *The Body of Life*

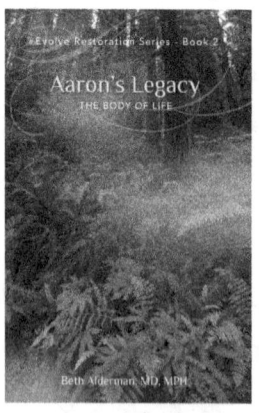

ISBN: 978-1-7321110-6-6

Having come to know the community, Aaron receives his legacy as a series of enactments of SIRC's history. The surviving members of his mother's old friendship group—Sarah, Doug, and John—join the audience and performers in processing and adapting their shared narrative. In the intervals between enactments, Rafa undergoes initiation while Aaron explores the composer, an instrument that enables a player to evoke memories with images and to express the player's responses as sound scapes. As Aaron shares his with Rafa, Sarah and others, John shares memories of Melissa, and seems to receive a new message from her.

As the community adapts to changes in its meaning and purpose, Rafa and Aaron each finds a first consort and draws inspiration from local knowledge keepers and change agents residing at SIRC, the nearby Monastery of Origins and Endings, or in Victoria or Vancouver. Aaron's health, damaged by his travel through a poison barren, deteriorates. With his death, his consort Parvati shares their legacy in the form of patterns of action that may remove roadblocks to continuous adaptation and renewal.

BOOK 3
The Kindred's Rebirth: *Rough Seas and Far Lands*
ISBN: 978-1-7332849-3-6

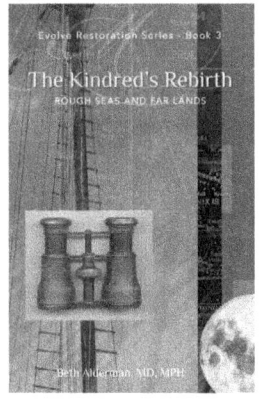

A decade later in Australia, Parvati and Björn give up on effecting meaningful restoration there. Dirk, while on his annual circuit of the north, arrives in Jokkmokk for the annual Sámi gathering to learn that SIRC is in crisis. Rafa, who is crossing the South Pacific on her two year global clinic circuit, hears strange news: the Fertility School, which was winding down, closed without notice. She realizes that her work, too, is drawing to a close as her clinics adapt to localism and begin to diverge.

All three travelers feel a strong homing urge and hatch a plan to converge in Scandinavia with the remnant of the SIRC community. En route, Parvati adopts a grandchild, Jacki, who helps Björn to recover from a disorder of interbeing. Many new consort pairs join the kindred and revive it by helping to form a next community, SIRC-Umea, and to organize and maintain residential restoration communities in the Baltic and North Sea bioregions, and to recover from the painful loss of the original community.

BOOK 4

Jacki's Vision: *The Green Line*

ISBN: 978-1-7332849-4-3

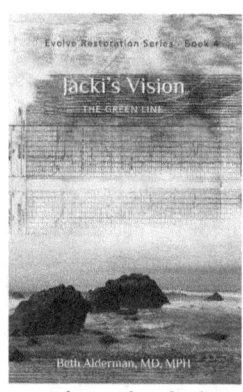

When Jacki turns sixteen, she begins her transition to adulthood by venturing into larger worlds of knowledge and adaptation to gain skills. During her first clinic circuit in the Baltic, she finds that her coming of age is coinciding with her kindred's restiveness. As she embraces and contemplates her future, a vision takes hold of her. She proposes a Green Line restoration project in Tasmania to reconcile a time debt created by the Black Line genocide, and to prepare her for organizing bioregional restoration projects. Her kindred and their networks embrace the project, expand it, and multiply its potential effects.

As the Green Line Corps prepares to depart en masse for Tasmania, Jacki meets a young stranger, Mirek, whose experience of the world—whose very umwelt—contrasts with her own. Later, in Tasmania, she gains a consort, Izaak, and a sister friend, Lally, both of whom winnow her possible futures. Together, the many thousands of Green Line participants develop a restoration ethos and synchronize living processes for restoring habitats—with their restorers. Jacki and her new peers are among the first to return to the original SIRC campus, near which many former kindred members have settled, and to which many others are about to return.

BOOK 5

Mel's Motherhood: *A Place in the Living World*

ISBN: 978-1-7332849-5-0

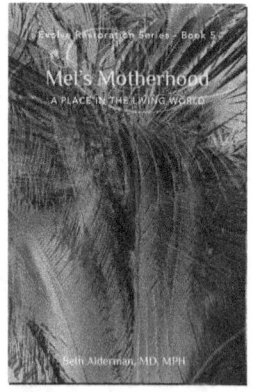

Mel and JJ—children of the Three Mammas—await the advance boat from Tasmania at the Cascadian Monastery of Origins and Endings. Mel, who is pregnant, and JJ, who fared poorly while he was away, finished their initiation projects and are keen to see Jacki and to meet the new kindred members. In the course of a joyful reunion, Mel and JJ learn that Jacki and Lally are also pregnant.

As this next generation of adults chooses ways to express fertility and defines new vocations, the reconstituting kindred celebrates new human lives, integrates with local communities, and processes hitherto hidden threads of SIRC's history with the aid of DNA fathers who participate. The complex, complementary communities adapt to continuous learning via phenomenology, and to continuous adaptation of systems for care and cure of evolved life.

Meaningful Retirement: *Become a Life Care Provider*

ISBN: 978-1-7332849-0-5

Meaningful Retirement is a self-guided monthly course in four seasons that can aid people like you who are exiting modern employment or withdrawing from the modern death economy. In it you will find a toolbox for transition to a vocation of life care, and thus begin to mature into a wise elder able to lead and mentor those who follow you. These seasons include:

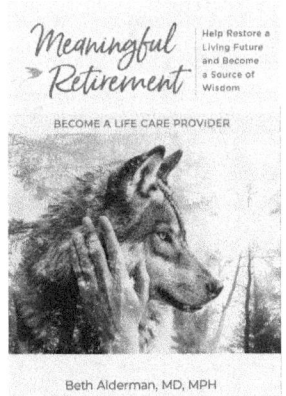

- **A Summer Breather**
- **A Fall for Reflection**
- **A Winter to Reclaim Your Personal Narrative**
- **A Spring for Revolutionizing Your Lifetime Learning**

As you transition to the role of provider of life care, you may choose to co-found emotionally and spiritually astute communities where you can mentor your juniors, who face the imminent and daunting task of passing through wrenching psycho-social change while arresting and reversing the accelerating human-caused Sixth Extinction. That threat to evolved life represents a unique crucible for transforming modern lifeways into ones that enable humans to choose and to restore life. Re-visioning and co-creating processes of care and cure that restore all lives as one will prepare your species to restore the planet's living lungs, its water circulation, its living shade, and its evolved resilience to unexpected planetary catastrophes. By viewing life in time though an eco-centric and eco-contextualized lens that scales from your lifetime to evolutionary time, you can begin to see your world through new eyes that reveal your place in the big picture of life on earth.

Direct learning, that is, phenomenology, is essential for restoration of a living future. This method has changed with every epoch since ancient natural historians began to attempt to create views, frames, and constructs in an attempt to grasp evolving generative systems. The present moment of peril can be taken as an impetus and inspiration to engage with an exciting process of learning and problem solving that some call the living paradigm. This paradigm, which is still incubating in fields as diverse as architecture and design, agriculture, archaeology, restoration, and theology, is ripe for grass roots syncreses across outdated fields of knowledge. When you learn to cooperate with the last hundreds of millions of years of evolution while pursuing space age ways of averting asteroid collision, you will be prepared to lead your species toward sustainability and to make room for rapid human adaptation that restores evolution. Welcome to the One Life..